Praise for *Choosing to Heal*

Janet Edwards's compelling account is empowering and informative for patients and health professionals alike.

Whilst being expertly guided through this topic in an empathic manner, the reader experiences a sound grasp of the topic with many fascinating insights into the patient's journey, treatments and outcomes pertaining to breast cancer in the modern National Health Service – and beyond.

This book is definitely one of the finest in this genre.

I sincerely hope that it will soon be found on recommended reading lists for students, patients or professionals involved in any aspect of this subject.

Dr Khalid Khan, General Practitioner and GP Trainer and
Tutor, Author of *Mnemonics for Medical Students* and
Medical Advisor to the International Journal of
Acupuncture. Fellow of the Chinese Medical Institute.

The title of Janet Edward's supremely helpful book says it all; we must act now and we must act fast to change the rapidly growing risk of breast cancer in the West. Janet has completely transformed her own experience of breast cancer, describing how she recovered her own health through her great creative intelligence.

Now, she seeks to transform our attitudes, motivating us to awaken from our passivity and say 'no' to the pandemic of preventable breast cancer in the West. We ignore this book at our peril, and I thank Janet whole-heartedly for bringing all the facts together in this powerful and elegant book which will change the lives of many.

Dr Rosy Daniel BSc MBBCh, Integrated Medicine
Consultant and Founder of Health Creation, Bath.

If I know anything at all about dealing with the shock of a cancer diagnosis, it's that the shock itself must be absorbed and acknowledged before radical procedures begin. Only then can the patient research for themselves all the existing options available and be in control of their own progress through the disease.

I honestly believe that the patient has to be on a par, almost ahead of their doctors at every step. Many doctors would disagree; Janet Edwards, the author of this invaluable book, would shout her agreement from the rooftops.

It charts her journey, both physical and psychological, through the minefield that was her own breast cancer and takes us through cause and effect in a unique way, treating us like the adults we are, rather than hapless bystanders.

In so doing, she illuminates the individual, holistic ways that cancer can be avoided and/or dealt with, if knowledge and, more importantly, self-knowledge are present. Yet, this is no flimsy, esoteric, alternative self-help manual. This is a cracking good read and should be a mainstream addition to the bookshelf of doctor, patient and curious layman alike.

Maureen Lipman, Actor.

Janet is a woman of extraordinary courage and charisma.

When told she was affected by cancer I absolutely had no doubt she would challenge it head on. She is one of the few people I know who could turn a negative into a positive.

By writing this book Janet will help and enlighten hundreds of cancer sufferers and answer the questions that they may be too frightened to ask.

With fascinating insight and empathy we follow her through a treacherous journey and come out the other end into a world of optimism. Janet cuts through the complicated jargon and makes cancer clear and comprehensive for everyone. She explores every avenue for a possible cure. We see her in both her confident and most insecure times.

Most importantly we learn how to deal with a disease whose name we are still sometimes too scared to utter.

This book will be a huge comfort and inspiration to those who read it.

Amanda Holden, Actor.

This book inspires other cancer patients to reflect before submitting themselves to the usual treatments which have only the destruction of the tumour as the goal.

At present there is no known treatment for the cause of cancer. Nobody can name the real cause as there are a thousand possibilities and therefore it is quite remarkable that nevertheless, very aggressive treatments are used. It is commonly acknowledged that in most cases these treatments do not work in the long term.

Like the author of this book, many people diagnosed with cancer try to find a new way which promises to tackle the cause, whilst not tormenting the organism with further problems as a result of the treatment.

The hypothesis of a lack of adrenaline as the cause of cancer, following long periods of stress in life, and a biological treatment developed from this theory, has been very successfully practised in my establishment for 50 years. In time, I believe this will continue to be proved scientifically.

The treatment is not expensive and so there is resistance from the cancer business and its worldwide economic interests. As a consequence, patients are deprived of the benefit offered by this non-invasive treatment.

Dr Waltraut Fryda, Cancer Specialist, Germany.

The multi-faceted musical abilities of Janet Edwards have long been recognized by so many theatrical and musical celebrities and performers, that one might not think it apposite, at first, to define her many talents.

From my own point of view, having known her for over 30 years, from the time my family first knew her as a brilliant and glamorous pianist, up until today, when she is an all-embracing musician, performer and teacher; all of her achievements have been successful and supremely productive.

As a professional singer, I worked with Janet in many varied Recitals, which were always rewarding joint musical experiences. Very soon Janet was able to bring her insight into teaching singers, across the board, to develop their talents, often in spite of strongly held biases and deep-rooted idiosyncrasies. Eventually, this led to a demand from well-known actors and actresses, to realise their musical abilities. This was not achieved without professional experience as her work as a solo pianist demonstrates. Her one-woman shows, many of them international engagements, were instrumental in bringing the regard which brought distinguished personalities to seek her advice and help.

Without doubt, the onset of cancer must have been profoundly shocking and disturbing for a busy professional woman, who had, throughout her wide-ranging musical career, been an equally busy wife and mother. The same application and tenacity that have always featured in her personal life were manifestly brought to bear in her disciplined approach to deal with this traumatic set-back!

Her desire to help others is demonstrated in her book so that the devastating effects of breast cancer may be ameliorated and fellow sufferers might cope by her example.

As she has taught many in the past to perform, learn, develop and progress, so now, she continues to rise to the challenge, offering the help that has been honed through her own life's experiences. I commend this book to all readers.

Dr Raimund Herincx B.Sc., AAIC., Hon D.Mus., Hon RAM.

Janet Edwards's account of her journey through cancer stands as a testimony to doggedness, optimism and the unbounded power of the human spirit.

It is also a convincing argument for the need for a mutually respectful relationship between doctor and patient working co-operatively towards health and well-being, an expression of a powerful belief in 'something more' than a mere mechanistic approach to healing, and an inspirational example of bravery in making critical decisions – some of them at variance with ruling medical conventions – based on her own intuition, research and experience.

I am privileged to have accompanied Janet on part of her challenging and moving voyage, and watched in admiration as she uncovered an important truth: health is not mere absence of disease, but a courageous, creative, ongoing process of balancing and re-balancing all aspects of our lives.

Garner Thomson, Neuro-Linguistic Programming ™
Meta-Master Practitioner and Trainer, Training Director of
The Society of Medical NLP™.

Changes in culture and in our environment always have consequences, and it is for us as humans to embrace the good and prevent the bad. This book describes uncompromisingly and personally how the rising incidence of breast cancer has become a tragic consequence of modern society, for which the causes have yet to be identified or any holistic cure found. Although we now live in a blame culture, in reality what is needed is for everyone to work together for the common good. In the front line, research scientists and clinicians need to turn greater attention towards identifying the causes of breast cancer, so that prevention might no longer be a confused dream but a reality. I hope that this book may provide a stepping stone towards this.

Philippa Darbre PhD, Senior Lecturer in Oncology,
The University of Reading, UK.

This is a bold and brave piece of work. The weaving together of personal experience, an exploration of the science and the discussion of cancer as a system disorder are indeed unique, and all in a language that can be easily understood. It should be read by every woman who has ever had any concerns about breast cancer … an enlightening read for both men and women.

Dr Nyjon Eccles BSc MBBS MRCP PhD
Medical Doctor and Scientist with Special Interest in Cancer.

Janet Edwards is a musician, teacher and composer whose performance career spans 30 years, from classical piano to musical theatre to soul, rock and pop. As a Neuro-Linguistic Programming Master Health Practitioner, she has explored the subtle connections between mind and body, using them to inform her own work and her students' training as well as her healing from cancer.

Choosing to Heal

Surviving the Breast Cancer System

Janet Edwards

WATKINS PUBLISHING

LONDON

This edition published in the UK 2007 by
Watkins Publishing, Sixth Floor, Castle House,
75–76 Wells Street, London W1T 3QH

Copyright © Watkins Publishing,
a Division of Duncan Baird Publishers 2007

Text Copyright © Janet Edwards 2007

1 3 5 7 9 10 8 6 4 2

Designed and typeset by Jerry Goldie

Printed and bound in Great Britain

British Library Cataloguing-in-Publication data available

ISBN: 978-1-905857-00-5

www.watkinspublishing.com

This book is not to be used as a substitute for professional
medical care and treatment. The ultimate decision concerning
care should be between you and your doctor. The information in
this book is offered with no guarantees on the part of the Author
and Publisher.

Contents

*This book is dedicated to the memory
of my loving mother Mary
and to those closest on my journey:
my husband Tom, and my sons Robert and Alex
who have unceasingly loved and supported me in
everything I have chosen to do.*

*I extend this dedication to all those men and
women who seek a way of healing the body
without harming it.*

Acknowledgements

My thanks to: Dr Waltraut Fryda, a truly holistic doctor who inspired me to write this book, for her wisdom, scientific knowledge and great ability to understand me that helped create my return to health. Dr Rosy Daniel, who set me onto the vital path which I might otherwise never have taken. Garner Thomson for his invaluable help in keeping me in touch with my essence – my instinct and intuition – and for writing the Foreword. John Baldock for his encouragement and his wisdom in editing my book. Dr Mostaraf Ali, Dr Wendy Denning, Dr Fritz Schellander, Robert Jacobs, Sue Kümmel, Dr Angelica Vogel and Dr Ingrid Giesow for being an indispensable part of the journey. My wonderful friends, Astra Blair, Katie Nouril, my cousin Daphne Harris, Aunt Alice, Svetlana Lazarevic, Anton Mullan, Helen and Tim Howland, Nicci Corrado, Jill Claxton-Oldfield and the many more who have continually encouraged me throughout. The brave and amazing women who contributed directly with their own experiences: Irene, 'Maisie', 'Ann', Linda, Sylvia, Pat, Diana and Patricia. Those who generously answered my queries whilst I was writing this book: Dr Waltraut Fryda, Dr Philippa Darbre, Garner Thomson, Dr Nyjon Eccles, Roger Coghill and Bill Sturgeon, and all those who endorsed the book including: Dr Raimund Herincx, Amanda Holden, Dr Khalid Khan and Maureen Lipman.

Thank you to all those who kindly gave me permission to quote from their publications which are acknowledged in the Notes section at the end of the book.

Foreword

Courage, as is often explained by many of those commended for extraordinary heroism, is not to act without fear, but to define and act on a deeply held conviction *despite* great – and sometimes overwhelming – fear.

When she received her life-changing diagnosis of breast cancer, Janet Edwards rapidly discovered that her conviction was that she was a whole person, deserving of respect and treatment as such, rather than simply the bearer of a disease over which she had no say or control.

To pursue such a conviction required true courage. Not only did she find herself engaged in trying to understand the alien and frightening process her body was undergoing, but also that her beliefs brought her into direct conflict with much of the research, and many of the ruling experts, of the orthodox medical world.

Unlike many other women who find themselves suddenly labelled as cancer 'patients', 'victims' or 'sufferers', she chose proactively to seek information, to bring to bear on the available data both her intuition as a creative artiste and her acutely developed critical facilities, and to make decisions, some of which ran directly counter to the medical advice she received.

Her book, *Choosing to Heal*, is her story, and stands both as testimony to her intellect, emotional depth and determination, and as a beacon of hope to other women now at the starting point of a similar journey.

But, even though Janet decided at a relatively early stage to stop traditional chemotherapy-based treatment and seek out a regenerative, integrated, yet still scientifically based, approach, this is no warm and fuzzy wholesale endorsement of 'alternative' treatments for a challenging and frightening disease. She submitted all claims – conventional or complementary – to the same, intense intellectual scrutiny, accepting some and discarding others that were not a match for her unique beliefs, values and needs.

Like Joseph Campbell's Hero's Journey, hers has been marked by significant calls to action, challenges and moments of decision. Her voyage has been rich in incident, discovery and insight.

For my part, it's difficult to decide which of these will prove most valuable to the reader, whether he or she is facing a similar life-threatening challenge, or is a medical professional open-minded enough to benefit from the solid, painstakingly researched factual information she presents.

Most impressive, I find, is her refusal to compromise her unshakeable conviction that we are more than a collection of functioning or malfunctioning organs and cells, and that we are an intricate open-ended psycho-biological system, part of even greater and more complex social systems, all in constant process of balance and change. Indeed, the belief that we can heal only by micro-managing disease, without regard to the macro-management of healing and health, persists in the largely Cartesian world of Western medicine. It is not only self-evidently and scientifically wrong, but, in many cases can be as actively death-dealing as the disease itself.

Equally important is Janet's understanding that the healing process should be a co-operative, mutually respectful venture with health professionals we trust. By taking responsibility for living a healthier, more proactive and positive life, we also need to be prepared to take decisions, some of which may run counter to the official party line. It helps if we can work with health professionals who trust us as they would have us trust them.

This takes real courage, not just because such a decision may prove wrong, but also because many medical experts are quick to label as 'heart-sinks' those patients who question them, or seek to expand their options. Janet is no Pollyanna. Her decisions were – and continue to be – made in the light of the best data available to her.

Janet's discovery that there are many health professionals who are fully aware of the limitations of the Western medical paradigm, but who are prevented by governments or insurance companies from following any pathways other than those that have their approval, is deeply significant. This book, far from the doctor-bashing so frequently indulged in by the alternative therapies, is as compassionate towards doctors' limitations and frustrations as it is to those faced by many of their patients, and stands also as a call for, and a contribution to, a new and more hopeful model of health and well-being.

The truth is that none of us can predict with any accuracy how long we have left on the face of this planet. We have little guaranteed control over when we die – but we do have complete control over *how* we choose to live whatever part of our lives is left to us. Science (with possibly most people) pursues longevity as a goal, with little attention to the quality of our daily life. It's sad that so many of us only pay attention to nurturing quality of life when that life is under threat, and even sadder, perhaps, that lifestyle management and enhancement are still regarded by many doctors and patients as largely irrelevant to the practice of health.

But, perhaps this is cancer's unexpected positive side effect. If, as we are often told, one in four of us will be affected by the challenge at some time in our lives, even the most recalcitrant defender of orthodoxy may one day be called on to face his or her priorities, values, and beliefs – and to focus, not on how to live longer, but on how to live well.

Since I have been privileged, personally and professionally, to accompany her on part of her journey, I can testify that Janet lives well. And the ambiguity is intentional. She embraces everything life has to offer with energy, enthusiasm, generosity, gratitude and love. She continues to learn, create and pass on to others the richness of her many gifts. By all the overt markers of health, of which joy is paramount, she *is* well.

Garner Thomson

Meta-Master Practitioner and Trainer of NLP
and Training Director of The Society of Medical NLP

Introduction

Several years ago, I set off with a backpack for the foothills of the Himalayas to find my grandmother's birthplace. On my travels I visited the area of Dharamsala in Himachal Pradesh, towards the borders of India and Tibet and the home of the Dalai Lama. One day, following a footpath up to the mountains, I came across a noticeboard and there, written by hand, was a statement saying that a young Tibetan nun had had her breast cut off by the enemy on the Tibetan-Chinese border. I was horrified at this hideous and misogynistic brutality. Little did I guess that a few years later I too was to have a breast cut off – not by enemy soldiers, but as part of the standard treatment for breast cancer.

There is a mistaken belief that surgery, chemotherapy and radiotherapy are 'state-of-the-art' treatments and apparently, because they are so good, all our hospitals are united in offering them as the only available treatments. Any treatment other than this is viewed by the medical establishment as being second-rate. However, it must be realized that the idea of this treatment always being the best is not borne out scientifically, and yet any other type of treatment is viewed by those in orthodox medicine as 'alternative' – a term commonly and erroneously understood as meaning not only second-rate, but also not 'scientific'. This flaw in our perception creates and perpetuates a treacherous myth. We are not seeing the truth. This fallacy is propagated by the medical establishment, the pharmaceutical companies and the media; but it is not the truth. The reality is a 'cancer business' endorsing a pharmaceutical-technical based training for doctors and the propagation of money, power and greed, which has grown into a gross un-truth.

Materialistic achievement has become the target. The sales of chemotherapy drugs in the USA alone, increased from $3 billion in 1989, to $13 billion in 1998.

In United Kingdom (UK), the 1939 Cancer Act continues today to bind doctors by law to offer only surgery, chemotherapy and radiotherapy as the standard treatment for cancer. The important fact, usually glossed over, is that normal orthodox treatments do not have the highest rate of success in curing cancer. Actually, the highest monitored rate of success belongs to the Gerson Therapy (*see* page 26) which, unlike more conventional treatments, acknowledges that cancer is essentially a systemic disease. A systemic disease is one that develops in the physical body over a period of time, and its successful treatment necessitates addressing the root cause or causes of the disease. It is not enough just to cut out the tumour, which is merely a symptom of the disease. There are other treatments which not only show high rates of success, but also equally high rates of non-recurrence. Because these other treatments do not abuse the body, the illogical fallacy appears to arise that as a consequence they cannot work successfully. Scientifically, it is clear that other methods allow our own highly sophisticated bodies to correct themselves. This is achieved by restoring the body instead of destroying both healthy and unhealthy cells which is what most of the current orthodox treatments do.

Dr Rupert Sheldrake, the eminent biochemist, Fellow of Clare College Cambridge and Research Fellow of The Royal Society, believes that science should 'start from experience' and that the much maligned 'anecdotal evidence' *should* be taken into account. We continually have evidence of this need as the Establishment drags its feet in the face of the many glaringly obvious problems that are brought to public attention through endless anecdotal evidence; mobile phones and the hazards of electromagnetic fields being just one of these issues. There is no point in science taking a 'holier than thou' attitude and ignoring the experiences of ordinary people when it is obvious that without this anecdotal evidence we would be at a standstill with very little, or no progress ever being made. Whilst scientific research can be a salvation to us, by its own admission it can also be riddled with flaws and double standards. It is time for us to pause and look at the reality: the present-day conventional treatment for breast cancer is not good enough. It is an extremely mutilating process whilst many of the new, so-called wonder drugs leave a trail of devastating side effects.

It is the scientific therapies that do *not* abuse the body that should be our foundation and the first call of research in curing cancer. There is no doubt that this is what people would prefer, given a choice. What has gone wrong? In our modern world of rapid communication, the range of choices and information on offer is greater than ever before, yet still we are being denied access to non-invasive restorative treatments.

These other treatments are not the only thing being denied. Somewhere in this gross myth, mainstream research into causes and prevention is also being denied. Scientists involved in this field of medical research are faced with a choice: they either live and work in collusion with this denial or – as many research scientists have already done – they leave to search for independent laboratories, sometimes going to countries where they can work free from these forces of denial, in pursuit of the truth.

In my own case I classically followed the conventional route of standard treatment in the earnest belief that this treatment must be the best, simply because it was given to everyone. Only when I had acquired enough information and observed myself in the process, did I hear alarm bells in my head. Then I realized that I had forsaken my whole understanding of the body as I knew it through my work, and could see clearly how the course of treatment was entirely at odds with my own philosophy. In my work as a professional musician and voice coach, helping and nurturing the voices of my students, I have learnt how important it is to care for the whole person. It is also important for my students to develop their self-awareness. One of the most important steps towards self-awareness is to listen to the body and still the mind until finally we can see ourselves as the amazing creatures we are. It is a vital part of our existence. Yet, as author Gilly Smith says:

> Our self-awareness about our physical and biological nature has been considerably weakened in modern Western culture. Our own bodies have become industrialized by the Industrial Revolution. We have internalized the Industrial system and the Industrial image in our minds, our psyche and our body. We have developed an arrogant anti-nature, anti-biological attitude through which we are disturbing the physical nature of the earth and undermining our own physical health and well-being. In our indiscriminate use of drugs and vice and environmentally injurious technologies, we are failing to recognize that we are part of nature. [1]

To be truly self-aware is a healthy state to be in since it protects us from many harmful situations, and so it is preferable that we do not wait until a crisis occurs before becoming self-aware. The problem of tackling things at the time of crisis, particularly in the case of breast cancer, is that the situation is often compounded with ancillary problems which tend to mask our true priorities, thus making the whole procedure more complex. So it is important to be fully aware and at our best when dealing with such situations. By doing this we build up our inner reserves in order to deal with all that life has in store for us, and it helps us to take a positive outlook during the inevitably difficult times. When first diagnosed with breast cancer most women do not feel ill and yet they are told in a very straightforward manner that they now have a potentially life-threatening disease. Naturally they are in deep shock and very frightened – and usually know little about what the procedures will entail. A woman who, in the course of her work, sees many women with breast cancer told me how profoundly aware she had become of the speed of the process and the lack of time given to women to fully understand what is about to happen to them. From diagnosis to mastectomy or lumpectomy and reconstruction, the process can be as little as two or three days, or one or two weeks. This is an exceptionally short time. Stunned, dazed and dealing with information overload, a woman is very unlikely to be making informed decisions – even though she is trying to make sense of all that is about to happen.

When we are faced with a huge, even life-threatening problem, our self-awareness needs to be extra sharp. Acknowledging that we cannot deal with this problem on our own, we need to carefully select and enrol others – perhaps the person nearest our heart, or in addition those whose wisdom and knowledge we value highly. It will be a time to select with all the precision we can muster, continually bearing in mind our goal, as we call on all our inner reserves.

Women facing breast cancer have very specific needs; needs which often can only be fulfilled by a very strong partner. I am not talking about the most obvious need, which is to be taken into the arms of a husband, lover or close friend – a woman must have plenty of that throughout her journey – but about having a person at the side of you to support you and to put a masculine energy into the questions you want to ask. Confrontation requires a masculine energy, and whether this comes from a man or a woman is irrelevant. This is the time when many questions arise and helpers are required to gather information and, if a woman prefers it, to stand up and speak on her behalf. Yet it appears that the present system of dealing with breast cancer is not always conducive to this for those who ask questions or seek different treatments. Above all, the patient must not be belittled or patronized. She should be made to feel at liberty to make her own decisions and know that she is totally supported by at least one person close to her. This is the time when compromise is not an option; you have to find the best for yourself.

Cancer doctor Rosy Daniel in an interview for the *Evening Standard* said:

... what disturbs me most about the orthodox approach

is the lack of emotional support for NHS cancer patients. These people want help. They have had a bombshell explode in their lives, yet doors are shut in their faces when it comes to helping them gain the will power they need to fight for their lives ... We are only just beginning to understand how powerful our body can be at healing itself, and also how precarious its nature is ... Conventional treatment, we should remember, is far from foolproof. [2]

Those of us in caring relationships, with or without children, married or not, young or old, will come up against difficulties along our journey, for many reasons. Illness is just one of them. It doesn't have to be severe or life-threatening for us to have to make changes in our lives and 'be there' for a loved one. If we are fortunate, it will soon pass and we can resume the easy, happy, loving relationship once again.

Many people might be forgiven for believing this to be the same for those who have had breast cancer – the so-called 'survivors' (a term I prefer to avoid) – and that these 'survivors' then resume their loving relationships and, enriched by this life experience, drift with their partners into the sunset years, a smiling couple in a truly Hollywood ending.

This is not the reality. The scenario might apply to a few relationships, but not the majority. The illness very often leaves an indelible mark on a couple, and the side effects of the treatments are capable of destroying many relationships when they are put to the ultimate test. Many men are unable to look at their wives' or lovers' wounds and scars, and are not even able to hold their women or talk about their breast cancer. On top of this, the woman may well find that the treatments have physically affected her relationships. It is possible that a young mother may not be able to lift her baby or young child, which can be devastating for both of them.

Following breast cancer, those women not already in intimate relationships often give up all hope of ever having a partner in the future. The very core of a woman's femininity has been dealt a cruel blow: a breast or a part of a breast has been removed – turning what is left of her into an uncomfortable, unfamiliar and distorted stranger. She feels incredibly vulnerable, unable to see herself 'whole' any more. Her predicament is made worse by the fact that breasts come cheap these days. In the 21st century we have truly realized the coming of age of the Barbie doll. If a breast isn't the 'right' shape or size, it is no problem to fix it. These are the new toys. In 2004, the most sought-after woman on the Internet in the UK was Jordan, the well-endowed celebrity glamour model. The 'Page Three Girl' and the acres of ample cleavage on view in photos of celebrities in the media, indicate that this is what we should be aspiring to. Where does this leave the woman newly diagnosed with breast cancer?

There are other women who see their breast cancer as something that modern medicine has conquered and who follow the prescribed course of treatment without query, attempting to push all thoughts about what is going on in their bodies or what might have caused this, to the back of their minds, resuming their lives after a very quick operation and reconstruction, as if nothing had ever happened. At least, this is what the medical establishment appears to hope for, as such an attitude conforms with the treatment they offer, which appears to be, 'There's something wrong. It is cancer. Cut it out. Hopefully make it look like it did before, then stitch it up and get on with life.'

Yet there is also evidence of a change of attitude amongst women towards breast cancer. What is happening and why? In spite of careers blossoming for many women, once a baby arrives it is the same for us all – our lives change. Having children is one of the most educational times for a woman when she begins to realize her capability to care and nurture. Looking after the health of her family is something that she moves into as a natural progression. She generates well-being – the antithesis of destruction. How can she then equate this with putting into her body the destructive carcinogens contained in many of the breast cancer drugs and in chemotherapy when she finds a lump in her breast, especially when she is told that she *must* do this if she wants to see her babies and children grow up? Furthermore, many of the treatments on offer may well rule out the possibility of having a first or subsequent child. This only begins to touch on the problem as she queries what the treatment is going to do to the rest of her body.

But questioning the treatment on offer is not enough. We also have to learn to protect ourselves against the increasing incidence of cancer, something unattainable as long as we live close to the boundaries of depletion and poor nourishment. Living in a fast-moving society, we may survive depletion in the short term, but it is highly dangerous in the long term. Organic diets alone are insufficient. Extra physical, mental and emotional activity requires extra fuel for all aspects of our speedy lives in order for us to become abundantly healthy and happy. Anything less and we open the door to degenerative diseases and depressive states of mind.

The more we all understand about breast cancer, the greater the likelihood of progress in the prevention and treatment of the disease. I trust the account of my own journey will help reveal and bring into focus some of the truth in this vast and complex picture, empowering not only women with breast cancer, but all men and women everywhere, to demand restorative and holistic treatments instead of destructive ones.

I hope that in my writing I am able to help some women to understand at least a few of the things that I have learnt in trying to unravel this strange journey, and that it might be useful to their own understanding and self-nurturing.

Part One of the book gives a simple outline of my own journey in which I eventually moved away from the standard treatment I was offered to another, essentially orthodox (not 'alternative') treatment to reverse the cancer. My diaries help to give a picture of the time I spent there. Part Two looks at the politics, the lack of research into cause and prevention and the unsatisfactory areas of the current screening and treatment of breast cancer. It also contains a questionnaire I compiled of frequently *unasked* questions for women who have or have had breast cancer, together with the response from a number of women willing to share their own stories. Part Three gets to the heart of the disease, how and why it occurs and what we can do to prudently avoid it. The environment, menopause and breast health are included in this. Part Four illustrates how I apply a holistic approach in my own sphere of work and gives the views of others involved in helping women with breast cancer. It looks at the heart of health, showing how we can empower ourselves to help prevent the disease.

If anyone can make the much needed changes in our attitude to breast cancer, it is we ourselves. It is you and I who must lead the way and not wait for committees, institutions and government bodies. It needs us to make the changes at a deep personal level in order to bring back a balance in our existence with nature and the world. It is the feminine aspect, the mother earth that has got lost and it requires us all, both male and female, to bring it back. We need the masculine energy of those good men – men of integrity – who have the balance of the feminine, effortlessly within themselves. These people, including the many good men and women scientists now at the leading edge of research, will be our greatest allies in making this happen. Some of these men and women are here in this book; out there are many more, compassionately searching. We must look to the past as well as the future without bias and dogmas, for the answers have always been there for us.

At some time in the not too distant future it would be wonderful if we could reach a place where no one would ever have to say again, 'There is something wrong, I am ill, and nobody is able to fully understand how to restore my health.' Then the disfiguring mastectomies and lumpectomies of the present day could be looked upon as primitive medicine, an act of barbarism belonging to the past.

PART ONE

A Personal Journey

The Great Integrity
is the physician of the universe
who heals without harming
and who acts without contention

Lao Tzu, *Tao Te Ching*

1 A Hit and a Miss

As a personal landmark, 2001 was unique. In September the Gershwin track *Jazzbo Brown* from my new CD, *Songs Without Words*, went to number one on the worldwide MP3 music server chart, whilst other tracks went into the Top Forty. Later that same week, I had a mastectomy for cancer in my left breast. Unique? Probably – and you could say, a rather strange autumn. It took two years for me to fully realize that my music had momentarily reached number one, for my mind had completely pushed this and almost everything else into obscurity as I began the most hazardous journey of my life.

Like all authentic myths and fairy tales, full of gallant knights and angels of goodness, the story was set through with villains and devils – often disguised as angels – and trials by fire, until I landed safely through the torment and the life-threatening situations. I was definitely not the 'heroine' type. Moreover, I was to discover that I was relatively naive in the ways of the world. I believed that living in AD 2000 meant that the world I was about to enter into on this journey was enlightened, seeking the good, and had done away with acts of barbarism – well, that's what we're supposed to believe – so it was natural to put my trust in it, especially as I was very happy with my husband, close family, friends, colleagues and my work with music: that was my life.

The heroines of mythical stories are given attributes and gifts to see them through their journeys. These gifts are sometimes acquired through the hardships they encounter in their lives, thus enabling the heroine to take responsibility for herself and make informed choices in her quest. The gifts often remain ignored until the heroine, awakened from her sleep, realizes that danger is not far away. So, true to the form of these stories, I remained only partly awake at the beginning of my journey, but a sense of taking responsibility for myself kept me awake enough to understand where I must begin looking. Like most people, I knew that if I wanted to sort out a problem, then the only way was to diligently uncover what was on the surface, and then search to the bottom. This is the way I work when I have to help fellow musicians with problems, so it was the most natural thing to do.

To make sense of this life-changing event, first I had to look back to the months before, delving into my diary to try and uncover anything that might help me to understand where this illness had come from, and in particular to appreciate that my instinct and intuition had been the only totally reliable factors in this unfolding story. Still very much asleep at this point, I began to use my intuition and instinct as tools to uncover the path I needed. So, the search began and the diary revealed:

January/February 2001

The beginning of 2001 had been extremely busy as I was completing my piano album and dealing with all the paperwork that goes into such a project. Permissions had to be sought from Universal Records for my 'spoof' piano arrangement à la Rachmaninoff and Mozart of Tom Jones's hit song *Sex Bomb*, whilst the Gershwin Trust in America had to give me permission to record *George Gershwin's Song Book*, Gershwin's own piano improvisations based on his songs. I had set myself a deadline to finish my own compositions for the album and to have a CD completed by the beginning of April, so it was a busy time as I worked on through the end of the winter of 2000 into 2001. The Gershwin music had served me well over the years, as I had performed many of the nineteen short pieces in my one-woman shows, cabaret and concerts; above all, I now wanted a completed recording to allow me to move on to new projects.

The final effort to provide Universal with the master recording for pressing seemed all consuming. By the end of February it was ready and I collected it from my sound engineer Dave Lewis at his studio in Bristol, leaving late that night with my husband Tom, to drive through thick fog to a hotel near Universal Records in Blackburn, Lancashire, where the recording was to be pressed. Weary, we arrived after midnight and rose early the next morning to deliver the master.

March 2001

On 1 March we were on a plane to Dubai for a much needed break. Dubai in the winter is a wonderful luxury – a combination of glorious weather, sunbathing and beach, with a bustling twenty-four-hour commercial life – a favourite place of ours with happy memories of the several concerts I have given there. All too soon the week had gone by and we were back home feeling refreshed, just in time to catch the last performance of David Hare's play *Skylight* directed by my old friend James Sykes at the Lawrence Batley Theatre in Huddersfield, Yorkshire, where some of my own music from the new album was being used for the play.

I followed this trip with an after-dinner talk and a short cabaret for the Inner Wheel in St Albans. A day or two later, thanks to Guy Fletcher at the British Academy of Composers and Songwriters, actor Jeremy Clyde telephoned to invite me to workshop a new musical of his called *What's the Score?* The music was written by Jeremy, with lyrics by David M Pierce, and the musical was devised and directed by Marie Macneill. It was to be staged and performed in London – just a week later – at the Fortune Theatre, Covent Garden, to musical theatre backers, directors and others in the industry. The small cast of four was made up of Jeremy Clyde, Una Stubbs, John Macneill and myself. I had a wonderful role, with some excellent solo vocal numbers, supported by a great band.

April 2001

To perform well, stage nerves can be an asset, consequently during *What's the Score?* I expected a healthy buzz of nerves before going on stage, but noticed something different. Although I could connect and perform well enough, somehow I wasn't getting the expected rush of adrenaline which made me wonder if I'd conquered my nerves completely. Only at the end of that year and after the breast cancer, did I look back and understand much more about why I wasn't feeling the 'buzz'.

Meanwhile, I had made an appointment with the dentist, as I'd been experiencing a lot of sensitivity in my teeth since our return from Dubai. A random X-ray revealed that a large filling was needed in my lower left jaw, so an appointment was made for a week or two later. At the same time, I was due for a mammogram test to be taken.

The mammogram didn't seem significant, as everything showed all clear. I hated the process, principally because it is such a barbaric way of treating the breasts. When I see my breast being put under great pressure in a translucent plastic press, it always reminds me of looking at pre-packed portions of chicken limbs in the supermarket. Not surprisingly, it is quite common for women to feel sore or sensitive in the breast for some time after the procedure. This was certainly the case on this occasion, and not for the first time. I returned to Wimpole Street to the specialist I'd used for some years and who had organized the mammogram, to be told that everything was normal.

Five days later, and back to the dentist to have the filling done. He commented that at my age it was unusual to need such a large filling as the really bad cavities had already been dealt with. Later in the year, as I began to understand more about breast cancer, I became aware that in Chinese medicine, which works with the network of meridians in the body, there is a specific meridian which runs from the particular tooth that was filled straight into the breast beneath.

May 2001

Anyway, all this seemed unimportant as we prepared for a happy event. Just a month after my mammogram, Tom and I took off for Spain as our friends Nicci Brightman and Giulio Corrado were to be married there. It was a truly beautiful wedding and also a moment to connect up again with colleagues in the music and theatre world. During our stay I had noticed a lump in my left breast, which had been very tender since the mammogram a month earlier, and wondered if the mammogram had disturbed a cyst, having had cysts occasionally before. We returned home a few days later and I developed a sickening headache and went straight to bed; but feeling worried about the lump, I telephoned my consultant who held a surgery nearby. He suggested that I went to see him straight away, so Tom drove whilst I sat in the back of the car armed with a bucket and all that was necessary for throwing up!

Within a few hours of our return from the glorious wedding and the Spanish sun, the doctor had examined me declaring that I had a cyst, which he understood was quite tender. Very concerned, I told him that somehow this lump felt different and asked how he could be sure that it was just a cyst. He seemed impatient, saying that I had only recently had a mammogram and 'no' he couldn't do an aspiration on the 'cyst'. It was at that moment that it suddenly flashed into my mind that his reaction could be something to do with not wanting to lose face with another professional, i.e. the highly regarded doctor who had read my latest mammogram test. He went on to tell me that I need not concern myself, as he could tell the difference between something that was nothing to worry about and something that was nasty. As we were leaving, he suggested in a rather brusque manner that I revisit him in three or four months' time. I had managed not to throw up in the few minutes we were in the consulting room, a great stroke of good fortune for everyone, and by the end of the day the sickness had stopped, leaving me totally drained. Tom suggested that I might visit a private general practitioner (GP) for a second opinion, but I said not, as it probably was just a cyst. In any case, the doctor had made me feel that I was making a fuss about nothing.

June 2001

The summer came: I felt tired and not ready to bounce into any new work. I had a few vocal students working with me and that was enough. There were signs of the rather late arrival of the menopause which seemed to be tied into the headaches and the sickness which had become a regular occurrence. The last big family party I had just given was for Tom and myself on our birthday in May (we share the same day). Normally I enjoyed cooking and entertaining, but now felt the need to ease off and let others lend a hand as I felt 'used up' and somehow needed to preserve my energy. This new outlook was probably the start of a healthy attitude towards myself, although I didn't realize it at the time.

July 2001

I was due for a routine gynaecology appointment and decided that this would be a good moment to let someone else take a look at the breast. By now the sizeable lump was bigger and my nipple was beginning to draw to one side and invert. At the examination the consultant observed what he called 'a thickening' around the lump, commenting at the same time that my breast specialist was 'a good doctor', and left it at that. Again I felt the condition was being brushed aside and that I was being given the 'we know best' pat on the head. I wasn't at all at ease with this, as again I was made to feel that this was nothing to worry about. Nevertheless I chose the easiest route, which was to accept their better judgements, keep optimistic and get on with life. A short time later on a lovely summer's day, I took a car journey to visit my dear friend Astra Blair in Buckinghamshire, continually having to adjust the car seat belt in order to avoid the discomfort and tenderness across my breast. I joked about the cyst as we chatted in the garden, saying that my left breast resembled the shape of an ashtray when I was lying down.

August 2001

I had a sense of waiting, lying low, reserving myself, rather like a creature in hibernation, whilst at the same time I continued to present my usual self to the world.

Although I had been told twice not to worry, at the end of the first week I was still concerned and went to see my friend the naturopath Robert Jacobs. After explaining my anxiety, he took a blood sample to send away for analysis to see if there was any sign of cancer. At about the same time I was surprised to receive a call from my breast consultant's secretary who, after a short while, realized that she was talking to the wrong patient, so rather fortuitously I took the opportunity of telling her that I was due for a check-up the next month, and so a slightly earlier appointment – in just ten days time, was arranged for 24 August.

Journey into the unknown: the initiation

At the appointment, the specialist immediately decided to send me back to the hospital for an ultrasound examination, where the doctor remarked that there was quite a change since the last visit and promptly did an aspiration into the lump. Now I was beginning to fear all that I had voiced at the beginning – that this was not a cyst – and on the evening of 29 August I took the telephone call which confirmed that the lump was cancerous. I felt numb with shock.

Suddenly, everything was on alert. It was late in the week and I had an ultrasound immediately on my liver, a chest X-ray and a scan of the ovaries, all of which seemed healthy; blood samples were taken and arrangements were already being made for the operation to take place on Monday, straight after the weekend. I was immediately plunged into an encounter with the unknown. What was going on? One day I am normal, and the next a surgeon is telling me that he will take this large, life-threatening lump – which was actually supposed to be cyst – out of my breast. My anger had not emerged yet as I was in total shock that the breast consultant was clearly ready to operate as soon as possible – not surprising when he'd thought that there was nothing wrong. Amazingly, in sheer fright, I agreed to the operation and then started to waken up to the full reality of the situation. I told Tom that I wanted a second opinion and we went for one straight away.

After an examination, our private GP thought I might well need a mastectomy and recommended that I go to the Royal Marsden Hospital in London, which is a National Health Service (NHS) cancer hospital with a private wing. There, at the end of the week, I saw Mr Sacks the breast consultant, who was sure that I should have a mastectomy. He said that he did not mind if I preferred to have surgery with my breast specialist as it could be done quicker, adding that he had spoken to him and had been told that it was unlikely the cancer would have spread to the lymph nodes. This was the first of many moments to come, when I was confronted with decisions that only I could make and none of them were what I had expected or desired. I was quite sure by now that I would never be seeing my breast specialist again. Knowing that he was not purely a breast specialist but performed other surgery, confirmed in my mind that I was right to wait a few days longer and have the operation with Nigel Sacks who suggested that I might want a reconstruction at the same time.

Whey! Hey! Not so fast! First I am told it is a lump that has to be removed, moments later it is a mastectomy, and now, at the same time I can have my breast 'reconstructed'! To many women, it must be an enormous relief to know that they can have a reconstruction straight away, and it appeared that the majority of women he operated on preferred this option. But to me this sounded as simple as ordering fast food and not the right thing to do. All I could think about was the time lost through misdiagnosis, and I knew that I could only cope with one thing at a time: just to clear the cancer seemed a big enough task. Then I realized that there was yet another problem that I must address. Being a pianist by profession, I knew it would be disastrous if I was not to have full use of my arm and, although I knew nothing about these procedures, I asked him to remove as few lymph nodes as possible and to take the greatest care.

The first challenge: surgery

September 2001

Tom dealt with most of the telephone calls that needed to be made and, although our friends knew that I was going into hospital, I chose to tell only a few of my closest students. The day before the operation I did a final, last-minute session with Amanda Holden who had an important audition which paved the way for her leading role in *Thoroughly Modern Millie* at the Shaftesbury Theatre in London's West End.

Waiting the few days until 7 September, the day I was due to go into hospital, seemed like a lifetime because in the back of my mind I had really been waiting since May. I rushed around to organize things, and the night before going into hospital Tom and I gave a ritual farewell to the breast which had fed my children and been such an important part of me as a woman. I was told that I might have to stay in more than the three or four days originally suggested and so, prepared with all that I might need, I arrived at the Royal Marsden Hospital at about two o'clock on Friday afternoon ready to be given surgery in the early evening. The private ward was very busy and we waited two hours whilst the previous occupant vacated the room which was to be mine. It was from then on that everything moved swiftly and I was soon being taken into surgery; I felt frightened, everything had happened so hastily and I even wondered if I would survive the operation, asking the anaesthetist outside the operating theatre to tell Tom and my sons Robert and Alex that I loved them.

I found myself back in my room one and a half hours later, attached to drips and drains. Tom was there waiting and immediately gave me some healing – one of the blessings and advantages of having a healer for a husband – and Robert and Alex were at my bedside. Thank God I was still here; the relief was enormous.

With excellent nursing, I was monitored continually and felt immobile for what seemed a long time, then gradually, over the next day or so I was able to go to the bathroom, attached to the tubes and bag containing the drain bottles; slowly I began to get myself together. There, looking in the mirror I first viewed the wound – a new flatness and a long cut where my breast had been. Even then I could not really say how I felt about the reflection in the mirror; I was too busy trying to understand all that was going on. I also noticed, to my surprise and alarm, quite extensive bruising around the side and just above the kidney area and was told that I had lost a lot of blood and body fluid in the operation, but fortunately had managed to avoid having a blood transfusion. My body appeared to have undergone a pretty large trauma and pathology was asked to take a look at my blood to see why the bleeding had been so extensive. My own gut feeling was that my body was in a state of shock, and that the bleeding was a reaction to it all. Mr Sacks remarked that in the circumstances it was better that I had not had a reconstruction and decided that I should be kept in hospital for a week, by the end of which pathology would know whether or not the cancer had spread into the lymph nodes. I had no idea at the time why some 21 lymph nodes were taken out, except that it appears to be standard procedure to remove quite a lot of them. Later, I learned that the lymph nodes help to drain away unwanted bacteria, dissolve the cancer and generally get rid of waste debris, so I wondered why the good ones should also be removed. If cancer is found in any of the removed nodes during subsequent biopsy, this indicates what further treatment may be required – usually chemotherapy. Obviously the number of nodes affected will vary, some women having many infected and others with very few or none at all. The number of nodes removed also seems to vary and this removing of the good with the bad, seems very wasteful.

Before the operation I'd been told to be prepared for some physiotherapy to help regain my arm movement. My ignorance was first-class at this stage and as I enjoyed tennis, practised Tai Chi and did plenty of walking, I viewed the forthcoming physiotherapy as if I were about to start a serious fitness programme! Post-operation, everything changed; firstly it would have been laughable to contemplate high activity with drain-tubes, bottles and bag attached to me as I trundled around, and secondly I was not feeling particularly strong. The physiotherapist gave me a few arm exercises to do, but I felt that these were insufficient and so, in addition, I began a gentle routine that Herman Chan Pensley, my Tai Chi teacher, had prepared for me of both pre- and post-operative exercises to further strengthen me, even though it was with restricted arm movement to begin with. Fortunately this gave me almost total movement before I left hospital and within a very short time of being at home the arm was back to full, normal mobility, which was quite miraculous.

With the operation over, I now needed to utilize the reading and research I had begun. Beside my bed was Professor Jane Plant's book *Your Life In Your Hands* which gave me her knowledge and views of breast cancer and told me what practical steps I could take to help myself. This and a first-rate juicing machine had been purchased just before the operation, thanks to the good advice of my friend Ali Stevens. Pain was not a problem, so I had no need for any medication for this, largely thanks to Tom's daily healing sessions which profoundly supported my recovery and well-being. The room soon looked like a florist's shop with bouquets arriving and taking up any available space, this being a tremendous boost to me as family and friends visited and helped me through the first week. My sons visited daily and Tom was with me at least once or twice each day, a pure labour of love, bringing food and fresh juices from home as he wholeheartedly supported my decision to aid my recovery through a new diet. At night, the room was far from restful with noise from the nearby Fulham Road, plus the additional problems of noise and light seeping into the room from the nearby nurses' station, which didn't make for a good night's sleep. I strongly recommend that anyone undergoing a stay in hospital takes with them earplugs and a sleeping mask.

The whole concept of the relationship between diet and cancer does not seem to have been taken on board by the mainstream medical establishment. During my stay in hospital I was offered all the foods which later I learned were detrimental to my healing process, and I asked to see a dietician as I'd clearly lost weight with the general physiological impact and trauma of the operation. It seemed to me, as I was finding through my continual reading, that diet is an important contributory factor to cancer, and I thought surely someone there in the hospital would be able to direct me. Our diet at home was always very good – lots of fish, some meat and plenty of fresh fruit and vegetables – but I needed more information in order to build myself up. It appeared that my request to see the dietician was unusual, but she duly arrived, sat down and listened to my concern about not wanting to lose any more weight as I was naturally quite slim. I asked her what I should do to try to gain weight. Her reply was simple; she said that I should try eating a few sweet biscuits. I was staggered at this, and felt it pointless to try and have any further discussion. However, it was just another eye-opener in my newly acquired understanding that despite being given good support from the surgeon, nursing staff and the breast care nurse, much of the medical establishment appears to be living on a different planet to most of its patients.

Deeper into the forest (and meeting obstacles with ever greater frequency)

In my case, and for most other people who have had surgery, there is an agonizing lapse of time whilst you wait to find out if the cancer has spread. Finally, the pathology results arrived to reveal cancer in three of the twenty-one lymph nodes that had been removed, and a grade two, oestrogen-receptor-positive tumour. Clearly the doctor who had diagnosed a cyst months before could not have been more wrong if he had tried. I was told that this would mean a course of chemotherapy, radiotherapy and tamoxifen and that I should begin as soon as possible. It was now mid-September which meant that by the following January, after chemotherapy, I should be ready for radiotherapy and then tamoxifen. It was much later on that I could see that I was in a state of shock, reiterating the words of the surgeon to my stunned husband and sons. Having nothing else to cling on to in this state, the surgeon's words were like a life raft and I took them with acceptance and determination. Maybe this is why so many of us go along with what the doctor says, rather than query it. Once the infection of the lymph nodes was officially recognized, I noticed a distancing arise from one or two of those who had been assigned to my case; there was a new seriousness in their attitude and at the same time I felt as if I was being kept at arm's length. I found this quite disconcerting to say the least.

For those who have witnessed the death of a relative or friend from cancer, it leaves a horrific print on the mind. It took many years before I was able to remember my mother as the beautiful woman that she was, and not the unrecognizable skeleton I had nursed through her slow death from leukaemia when I was 17. Afterwards, I reacted with a very positive effort to make something worthwhile out of my life. With huge energy I had thrown myself into carving out a successful career in music, getting married and having two wonderful sons – all with a full determination that I would not get cancer. Now I had to try to make some kind of sense out of everything that was happening to me. Naturally, my first reaction was that my own sons must be spared a similar terrible experience, and at all costs I must survive for my loved ones as much as for myself. How wrong it all seemed to be going at that minute when I was told to go home, and be ready to start chemotherapy in two or three weeks' time.

Following in the footsteps

Totally shaken, I could only think of my aunt, my mother's sister who, at around 60 years old, had had a mastectomy and was now in her eighties. It gave me hope in some way. At the time, she had been given a treatment which she believed to be an early form of tamoxifen, producing some unpleasant side effects. When she developed symptoms of septicaemia, her GP stopped the medication. There was no sign of cancer in her lymph nodes and she never had radiotherapy, so her situation was different from mine, but somehow it helped to know that she had survived her ordeal with surgery and little else. One change she made to her daily routine was to drink more water – only bottled water – from then on. Later, I learned that she was not happy about having mammograms and had refused them in recent years.

Somewhere during my trauma and uncertainty I began to notice how I really felt about what was happening. I realized a part of me feared chemotherapy, but not for the obvious reasons such as the sickness, and having to endure physically and mentally the process of all six sessions. I reckoned I could be 'brave' and believed I could be strong enough, but something else was happening. For some unaccountable reason, I found myself saying to Tom that I wasn't sure my body could physically take it and that these feelings were certainly not feelings of avoidance. It was a strange time, like a slow awakening. It was much later, looking back, that I could see it was the start of a long climb to reclaim the core of my being which somehow had been subtly slipping away.

Before I left hospital I had expected to see an oncologist to discuss the forthcoming treatment, but no one came, so it was left that the appropriate department would get in touch with me when I returned home. After some days and still no response, I rang the hospital, pointing out that I had been told that I should begin treatment very soon and yet I still did not have the name of the doctor who would be looking after me and dealing with my treatment. After much prompting I was given an oncology appointment towards the end of the month.

2 The Fog Descends

When I had asked the doctors whether there were any alternatives to chemotherapy, the answer was a resounding 'no'. I was told that the statistics for people who did not follow through the suggested course of treatment showed a low survival rate. There was a final, throwaway reference to the fact that – very occasionally – a person would have surgery and never return to the hospital for further treatment, and yet still survive. It was made clear that the chances of that happening were minute.

Back home, what now?

Mid-September 2001

Once home, I began my quest to find out what I could do about trying to help myself into a state of wellness. I was still in shock at the speed of things, the trauma of surgery and was feeling somewhat left in limbo. I quickly became more informed about cancer and after reading an article by Doctor Ali, who has a practice at the Integrated Medical Centre in London, close to where we live, I decided that although he had a long waiting list, I would just turn up at his surgery and sit there until someone would let me see him; I was not disappointed. The receptionist told him of my plight and he called me in to see him between appointments. I shook his hand, thanked him for seeing me and with blatant bribery, handed him a copy of my CD, whilst apologizing that I had just 'hijacked' his reception area. He listened carefully, then suggested that, although he couldn't say for certain, I might do a little chemotherapy and radiotherapy, but in general, not too much. The words 'not too much' resonated well with me, it felt prudent. He suggested that the next step was to make an appointment to see his colleague in the practice, Dr Wendy Denning. Apart from being kindly, he made lighter of my condition than anyone else so far and clearly saw my deep concern when he looked me in the eye, smiled and said, 'You've only got breast cancer,' as if I should be thankful that it was nothing more. Strangely enough, this was what I had needed to hear as somewhere a part of me was able to say for the first time, 'Take a breath, you can deal with this.' This liberation was so great that I left the surgery and found a secluded doorway a couple of streets away where I crumpled up in the entrance like some vagrant and for the first time, with great relief, tears slipped down my cheeks as I cried about the whole crazy situation. At that moment, I gave the doorway a six-star rating, it was better than the Ritz.

Feeling empowered for the first time, the next step was to visit Dr Denning as soon as possible. Here I began to see a fresh outlook to dealing with breast cancer. She ran tests to show the present status of my blood and what supplements I might need, and also recommended me to have vitamin C infusions to help deal with the effects of chemotherapy if that was the path I chose to follow.

Meeting the oncologist

Next, Tom and I went to my appointment with the oncologist at the Royal Marsden. I had a list of questions for him as I was not convinced that chemotherapy was the answer. Even now, I cannot remember any response giving me a clear indication that chemotherapy was greatly beneficial. The oncologist's figures, percentages and so forth were somehow vague, as were the possible side effects: however it was the only treatment of choice offered at the hospital. At this point the haze around me had grown thicker. Surely, I reasoned, it must help in *some* way, and any help, however little, must be an advantage, despite the side effects – which also included losing my hair.

What was the success rate of destroying the cancer by having chemotherapy? Figures of 10 to 15 per cent did not sound great but it seemed to be something. What other course of action was there? Simple – none. What about other therapies available rather than chemotherapy? Simple – none would do any good. I had shown concern regarding my high levels of oestrogen, so my next question was about tamoxifen as it was a standard medicine given to patients with oestrogen-positive tumours. Wouldn't it help to be taking it now rather than in several months after all the other treatments? The casual answer was that I could do that if I wanted to, which didn't seem like a rational, scientific decision on the oncologist's part, but rather one to keep me happy. Anyway, I decided to start the tamoxifen, although if I am truthful, not without putting it off for a day or two before taking the plunge.

This was the first time that I had ever been to a doctor to query my medication and when it should commence, and already, to my amazement it seemed that I could do whatever I wanted. Nothing was obligatory, despite the fact that we were dealing with a life-threatening disease; the decision was to be entirely my own.

The oncologist recommended a course of six chemotherapy treatments and said that if that proved too much, then we might stop them before the end. 'Proved too much', sounded like an exploration into the unknown, and highly distressing since it concerned my health. As my mother had died from leukaemia, I asked if there was any chance that the chemotherapy might also make me more vulnerable to getting it at some later time. 'No', was the answer, although I had read differently. He could see that I was not too happy about all this and suggested that I think about it and in the meantime he would make arrangements for the chemotherapy to begin the following week, on 2 October. The plan would be one session of chemotherapy in the day ward, then three weeks off to recover before the next session. If I didn't want to start so soon, then I could postpone it and begin when I felt ready. It all felt so uncertain and not a route that I had ever envisaged; but then I'd never envisaged getting cancer either. All in all I was feeling quite 'at sea' with everything.

The most disconcerting thing was the impersonal communication. It was rather like a brief interview with a college career advisor to decide on your life's vocation. Basing its guidance on the results of your exams, the college points you towards the course it thinks it would be best for you to take. What the college doesn't seem to offer is the course that is suited to one's individual needs. This, we are told, is not the point. These are the courses available. There is nothing else, so take it or leave it. Conform, or forget it.

I'm learning fast

The following few days were agony. By now I was also seeing Dr Rosy Daniel, former Medical Director of the Bristol Cancer Help Centre, who had huge experience of all these things and was to be my most valuable help in the months to come. On discussing the chemotherapy issue with her I clearly remember still not being certain about my decision. 'Wouldn't any help be better than none?' I asked myself. I discussed it also with Dr Denning and the breast nurse at Breast Cancer Haven in Fulham, London – a wonderful place offering complementary therapies and helpful advice to people with breast cancer – but realized that only I could provide my own answer.

I did not know it at the time, but doctors are not allowed to give their opinions, they can only give facts. It is therefore most important that you ask the direct question 'Would you personally have this treatment?' or 'Would you recommend this treatment to your mother, sister, brother etc. …?' (Not guaranteed to work, but it could help to build a bit more heart and feeling into the conversation.)

At this moment, I felt that I had fully enrolled and was well into the academic term of a degree course in 'How to survive cancer, hopefully without getting your fingers burned'. Earlier in the year, before I knew I had breast cancer, I had met psychologist Hertha Lareve, who also worked at the Bristol Cancer Help Centre.

She was a woman of great integrity who I felt might be able to be helpful to me in some way at this moment. Hertha had introduced me to Dr Daniel and also to Essiac, a herbal tea concoction of great help to cancer patients, available through the Clouds Trust charity.[1] Whilst trying to come to a decision as to whether or not to do chemotherapy, I brewed my first batch of Essiac.

Essiac

In the 1920s head nurse Rene Caisse, who was working at a hospital in Northern Ontario, had noticed an elderly patient with extensive scar tissue on one breast and discovered that thirty years earlier the woman had been diagnosed by doctors as having advanced breast cancer. Rene Caisse in her own words reported that the woman said, 'A very old Indian medicine man had told me I had cancer but he could cure it.' The Indian had then given her a tea made of herbs, one of which was sheep sorrel. Dedicated, Rene Caisse went on to experiment and recreate this tea and also produced an injection of sheep sorrel to give to cancer patients. Her rate of success for these patients was very high; however, despite many eminent doctors approving and encouraging her work and research, she was not allowed a licence to conduct her clinics unless her work was officially 'approved'. By 1936, after several unsatisfactory meetings with the Canadian Medical Association, she realized that it was unlikely that her successful treatment would remain available to cancer patients if the formula were to be turned over to some anonymous, large pharmaceutical company. She resolutely 'refused to divulge the Essiac formula until the medical profession formally recognized it and her work.'[2] Just before she died aged 98, she gave a version of her formula to the Resperin Corporation of Toronto for the sum of one dollar. She knew that this was unwise, but didn't want to die without passing on the formula. Sadly, and rather as expected, none of the proposed and promised trials were ever followed through. Now, by obtaining and brewing the herbs available through the Clouds Trust, it gave me some hope and encouraged me to begin to positively help myself.

Taking the plunge

Having gained further understanding of my condition, my big fear behind all that was going on was that my oestrogen levels were still very high. Although my periods were just showing menopausal signs of irregularity, the fact was they were still arriving roughly every three weeks. On average, I should have stopped having them altogether, but they seemed endless. Now, after the impact of surgery, I was frightened that unless they stopped soon, I would be further depleting my body's natural resources and this was something I felt I could not afford to do. The idea of the ablation of the ovaries sounded barbaric, particularly as I had avoided having a hysterectomy, being suspicious of drastic surgery unless it was vital. Neither was I in favour of taking hormone replacement therapy (HRT), as artificial hormones had health risks attached. I knew that just maybe, the chemotherapy would eventually stop the periods, as most women by my age were post-menopause. There seemed to be far too many really important things to think about all at once, and I found it absolutely exhausting.

Three days later the first chemotherapy session was due and by now I had decided that I must do it. I couldn't put my hand on my heart and say that I was totally sure about it, but still I was in a state of fear and confusion about 'not doing the right thing'. The actual physical side effects that I was preparing to deal with were not my main worry, although I certainly had no illusions that it would be easy. However, I voiced my fears to Tom, saying again I wasn't sure that my body would stand up to it. Well, I would give it a try; after all, the hospital had recommended that I do it. I was beginning to be aware of a gulf growing between the authorities who appeared to be responsible for my health and my own intuition and gut feeling. Still I was not prepared to 'rock the boat' and more willing to give the authorities the benefit of the doubt.

3   A Treacherous Path

Beginning of October 2001

For some time now, there has been growing awareness throughout the world, both amongst the general public and many in the medical profession, that chemotherapy could thankfully be abandoned if we were offered better, harmless and readily available alternatives. So what is it that still drives the majority of us, at a time when we are at our most vulnerable and alone, to accept this 'therapy' rather than searching out and taking another route? Just days before my treatment was due, I was still examining all that I had been told.

Clouded, gloomy and desperate to do what was best, after talking things over with Dr Wendy Denning and Dr Rosy Daniel I decided I would go through with it. It was totally my decision. The day before I was due to begin, I delivered some music to the Cambridge Theatre where *Fame* was currently showing and met up with my old friend, the musical director David Beer. As we parted he said encouragingly, 'Well, you have to give it your best shot.' I had to agree, by now I'd arrived at much the same conclusion.

Into chemotherapy

I opted to be on my own for the first chemotherapy treatment. It was to be one session every three weeks and a total of six sessions over a period of 18 weeks: after that, radiotherapy. Tom took me to the Royal Marsden private day unit, a rather drab-looking place with a room with armchairs all around the perimeter and a partitioned-off office where the nurses were stationed. He left and I sat down at 9am and waited for a nurse. It seemed that nobody knew who I was and had no record of my appointment. Eventually a doctor came, went away, and after a long time returned to tell me he had found my records and that he was the doctor who would be overseeing my treatment for the course of the day. I had never met him before and was concerned that he might not know my background, having discovered whilst reading Professor Jane Plant's book that people had died from being administered the wrong dose of chemotherapy. As no one seemed to know who I was at the beginning of the day, I decided I must check – as far as I could – that everything was properly in order before the treatment began.

The nurses seemed busy with everything except me, and as lunchtime got near I was no further ahead than at 9am It was suggested that I go for lunch and return later, but first I had to be weighed. By now I had learned that the chemotherapy drug dosage is based on the weight of the patient and so I asked the young nurse, who appeared to be the one who would administer the chemotherapy, if I should undress before being weighed. She said it would not be necessary, but I should take my shoes off. I had an uneasy feeling this would not give an accurate reading of my weight, but the fact that it was the usual routine – plus her reassuring smile – seemed sufficient.

Although, beforehand, I had found out what my therapy would be – standard breast cancer treatment with fluorouracil, epirubicin and cyclophosphamide (FEC) – in retrospect, again my naivety was colossal. I struck up a conversation with a pleasant woman patient who told me she was receiving a new chemotherapy drug as part of an experiment. I remember remarking how nice her hair looked to which she replied, 'Oh, it's a wig': she had lost her hair some while ago during the treatment. I quickly realized that if a patient looked as if they had come from the hairdressers, inevitably it was a wig.

By the afternoon, my chemotherapy had arrived from the pharmacy; everything was ready and so we could begin. First I had to thoroughly wet my long hair (cut a little shorter for the event) as I was to wear an ice cap to prevent me from losing my hair. The idea is that by drastically lowering the temperature of the head, this causes the blood vessels to dilate to such an extent that it protects the hair from the effect of the chemotherapy circulating in the blood. In an armchair nearby, another patient was receiving her final treatment from the senior nurse and wearing a huge cap which looked like a white cake.

The young nurse arrived with my ice cap. This was different: it was blue, rather like a jockey's cap, with a strap fastening under the chin, identical to the one another patient was wearing. The nurse attempted to put the cap on me – uncertain about how to get my hair into it. Apparently this was a new experience for her as these caps had only recently started to be used. Finally, after going off to consult with the senior nurse who was busy attending to the patient with the 'white cake' cap, she returned and began tucking my hair up into the back of my cap. It was not a great fit. She appeared uneasy and left the strap hanging loose, instead of fastening it. I was warned the ice cap might feel so cold that it would hurt my head for a short while, but it never did as it wasn't fitting tightly and the crown of my head was not touching the top of the cap. My nurse had another word with the senior nurse but made no further adjustment. Shortly after this, as the woman with the 'white cake' cap left the ward, I could see that her short hair looked good, except for the front which was a little thin. She was about my age and had undergone six sessions. This seemed reassuring.

The chemotherapy was brought over and after checking my name was on it, the nurse put the drip into my arm. She sat beside me to control how fast it went in and asked me to let her know how I felt and if I had any strange sensations. With my free arm I held the ice cap down in an attempt to get it to make contact with the top of my head. Shortly after the process began I felt a sensation around my sternum: the nurse smiled knowingly and said, 'You mean like heartburn?' I didn't ever recall having heartburn so I didn't know what it was like; anyway, she said that it was quite usual to feel this. Then suddenly, I began to see my anatomy as if I was working with one of my students, realizing that the place where I felt the sensation was in the area of my thymus – the heart of the immune system. An alarm bell rang inside me heralding a wake-up call.

A slow awakening to my precarious state

This was the first moment of seeing the connection of my life's work to where I was physically and mentally at that moment. The subtlety and sensitivity that I had used in helping to develop and restore people's voices was as far away from me as anything could be right now. This drip of chemicals was going through my system and neither I, nor anyone else, knew what the effects would be at that moment. For the first time I had truly opened my eyes to realize what I was doing. In that same instant my instinct was to stop the treatment, but I literally 'held on to my hat' and after 45 minutes I was through it. The drip was taken down and the senior nurse told my young nurse to inform me that at the next session, my hair should be left to hang beneath the cap and not tucked in. (I was to discover why later on.) I got my things together and went home armed with anti-sickness pills.

As I went to bed that night I felt a little nauseous, but managed pretty well until the next day when I began to feel rather tired. My period stopped abruptly within a few hours of having chemotherapy, and from that moment on never returned again. Over the next few days I felt low and tired – nothing surprising as I was ready for some sort of reaction.

The aftermath

I had made an appointment with a counsellor who had been recommended to me, as I realized that I needed all the help I could get
to overcome the cancer. The woman who was to help me was
kindly, but somehow did not seem right for me. I had experienced
therapy many years ago, and at the time the process had been one
of self-revelation and very important to me, setting me on a new
path during what otherwise would have been an impossibly
difficult time. What I was experiencing now was different and none
of it bore any relevance to my present situation, the chemotherapy
having taken place only two days before. I felt that a much more
sensitive and considerate approach would have been better.
However, it turned out that my being there did have a purpose – as
I was leaving, the counsellor kindly offered to lend me books and a
video which became very important to me.

The books were by Max Gerson, famous for his Gerson Cancer
Therapy. In brief, he acknowledges the low immunity and tissue
damage of a cancer patient and it is through his regime of a special
diet, raw fruit and vegetable juices, supplements, special injections
and enemas, that the body is returned to normal and the patient
free from cancer. In addition, the video *Cancer Doesn't Scare me
Anymore* by Dr Lorraine Day, Chief of Orthopaedic Surgery at San
Francisco General Hospital, was a colossal revelation. When Dr Day
had been diagnosed with breast cancer, she was recommended the
conventional course of mastectomy, chemotherapy and radiotherapy. She refused and overcame her cancer with a method similar to
the Gerson Therapy. In addition she had chelation therapy – a
treatment often used for unblocking arteries – which cleanses the
system, unlike the poisoning destruction of chemotherapy. Filmed
sitting at the desk in her office, Dr Day's non-stop commentary
was riveting. As she exposed the hypocrisy in the pharmaceutical
industry, she tore apart everything to do with the conventional cut,
poison and burn (CPB) cancer treatments. Laid before me were
facts instead of the twilight half-truths: dodgy statistics were no

longer part of the scenario. It was clear that there *was* a way through the maze. Thankfully, the counsellor who had given me this valuable information had provided me with the means to further empower myself in understanding cancer.

Unforeseen problems and no answers

A day or two later my cousin Daphne, one of my greatest supporters, came to see me and we went for tea at the local café. It was the slowest walk I have ever made and we both knew I was knocked out badly with the chemotherapy, but more was to come. That night I awoke to visit the bathroom and found I couldn't open my eyes. It was the most awful and strange sensation; my eyelids were sealed. There were signs of mild conjunctivitis, but this was not the reason they wouldn't open. The problem felt internal to the eye as if the muscles had completely shut down and I could only open my eyes with great effort and the help of my fingers. I returned to bed, only to have the same thing happen again when I awoke the next time. This was by far the scariest thing that had ever happened to me. Feeling ill or sick was to be expected, but this was different. Nobody had warned me about this and it was not mentioned in any of the literature that I had read. Although it was not painful, my body was no longer under my control and that was truly frightening. The same thing happened every night from then on, and in addition, I began to get a sore throat and felt worse over the following days. It was near the end of the second week so I hoped things would improve quickly as there was only one week to go before the next chemotherapy treatment. Meanwhile, to counteract some of the detrimental effects of the treatment, I went to Dr Denning at the Integrated Medical Centre for what was to be the start of a course of vitamin C infusions, and in addition, received healing sessions from Chris Howe.

Instinct and intuition surface

By now I had thoroughly looked into the previous blood test results and began to understand much more about the state of my body. During the whole of this period, from the moment I had started reacting to the chemotherapy, my self-awareness was growing and my instincts and intuition were surfacing rapidly.

At the end of the second week, worried about my sore throat, I called the hospital's chemotherapy day unit on my way to a support group meeting at Breast Cancer Haven. It seemed a good idea to visit a support group where I could share my experiences and concerns with other women and learn more about what was turning out to be this very strange journey of breast cancer. I arrived a few minutes late and quietly joined the circle of some eight to ten women. One young woman was noticeably without hair except for a few strands on top. As I sat down, a middle-aged lady was speaking: she was complaining about the people where she worked. She knew they were taking time off for no good reason, whilst she was faithfully at her desk each morning before nine, despite feeling desperately ill from a recent shot of chemotherapy. I noticed that there was a continual slight shake in her hand and her general appearance was that of a very unwell woman. I felt concerned for her and thought how lucky I was to have Tom and not to have to get up for work each day. Just at that moment my mobile phone rang, I had forgotten to switch it off and so I immediately left the room. It was the doctor at the hospital day unit who said that I must go there immediately as it was clear from my message that I had an infection. As I was finishing the call Louise, the nurse appointed to me at Breast Cancer Haven, came out of the group meeting to see if everything was all right. I told her about the infection and that I was not happy with my blood test results. She was sympathetic and could understand my anxiety, which further confirmed my feelings that things were not right.

I need answers

I immediately left for the hospital and on arrival met the doctor who had been on duty at my chemotherapy session. Clearly I had an infection. He took a swab from my throat and I asked if he thought it was bacterial or viral. The question seemed to be irrelevant to him and I was given a prescription for hefty antibiotics (I could not recall the last time I had taken antibiotics as it was so long ago). He told me to begin immediately in order to be ready for the second chemotherapy treatment the next week. When I suggested that it was very early in the treatment to get an infection, he shrugged his shoulders and said that it could happen that way. I told him of the problem with my eyes: he said it must be some sort of conjunctivitis. I told him that the mild conjunctivitis had cleared, I no longer had the symptoms, emphasizing that what I was experiencing was very different; I couldn't move the muscles in my eyes. He replied that he didn't know what it was – but probably it was conjunctivitis.

Enough was enough! At this point I decided that it was time for *me*, and me alone, to take charge of my life. I had no idea what I would do, but I knew to the core of my being that I was right. Logic stepped in alongside all the information that I had devoured over the last few weeks. I asked to see my blood test results. He took me to a windowless room with a computer – definitely not 'a room with a view'. There we sat at the computer screen for about an hour and I expressed all my doubts about chemotherapy being the appropriate treatment. I talked about my understanding of the subtleties of the body, gleaned from many years of work as a musician and particularly working with singers. I voiced huge concern over the fact that my eyes were not functioning properly and that the idea of this being made any worse by a second dose of chemotherapy was unthinkable. Finally I pointed to the low neutrophil count on the screen in front of us. I asked him at what point it was considered unsuitable to give a patient another dose of chemotherapy. The range of figures he produced included my current status: I pointed this out on the screen. He laughed and quickly reassured me that I needn't worry as my blood count would be back up by the next week because of the antibiotics I was about to take. Instantly I said how unsatisfactory it was that my treatment was to rely on antibiotics to get it started. To me it looked like a dangerous game of numbers and 'cooking the books' to fit the medical guidelines. There was nothing else left to say except, 'Forget it, I'm out of here.' I picked up my things and left. He said he would inform the oncologist of my decision and that I should phone if I changed my mind.

Determination to find a better way

The next day I threw away the booklet on hair loss knowing that I would not be returning for any more chemotherapy. For the first time I felt sure of myself, as if a great burden had been lifted. I took the antibiotics and responded well, but still my eyes would not open during the night. The following week I attended an oncology appointment with Tom, who had been totally supportive of my decision. Tom had seen first-hand, the devastating effects of one dose of chemotherapy, and knew it was wrong. At the meeting the oncologist made it clear that there was no alternative treatment and that I would not be able to go back to chemotherapy if, in the future, I changed my mind. Again, he could not explain my eye condition and the meeting left me with a feeling of abandonment. Fortunately I was now ready and fired up to actively seek out a way to nurture my immune system, instead of annihilating it. It was understood there was to be no further chemotherapy and consequently my appointment for radiotherapy was brought forward. From now on, I was determined to have a *complete* understanding of any possible treatment that I might consider.

I was not alone, I had the support of Tom and Dr Rosy Daniel; without them it would have been much more difficult. A few days after the oncology meeting I had an appointment with Rosy and told her of my decision; she had no difficulty accepting that chemotherapy was finished, and that now self-nurturing was the way forward. With her help I knew that I could monitor my condition and embrace the search I needed to make in order to restore my body to good health. It became impossible to talk about my attitude towards chemotherapy with those people who adhered to what I considered by now to be the somewhat dangerous gospel of 'do only that which your doctor tells you to do', as I found their comments disempowering.

Some weeks later I had a routine check up with Mr Sacks, the surgeon. When I told him of my decision to discontinue chemotherapy he commented that chemotherapy doesn't suit every body. My feeling was that as this is certainly true, then it means that the treatment is an 'experiment' for every individual, and, as I had already been told by my oncologist, no alternative was available.

Furthermore, Dr Allen Roses, worldwide vice-president of genetics at GlaxoSmithKline, admits that drugs used in the treatment of cancers are effective in only a quarter of the cases.[1] As my research progressed, I found others who believe the figures are worse. No one knows how great the cost might be of the side effects of treatments, which may reveal themselves immediately, or in years to come. Generally, booklets on chemotherapy have a section on side effects, one even stating in bold print: 'However, sometimes there may be permanent damage,' and 'If this is likely, your doctor will discuss it with you before the start of your treatment.' How can your doctor be certain there will not be damage and possible permanent or long-term side effects, which include damage to the heart and secondary cancers? I was told by a member of staff at one of the cancer telephone helplines that five years is considered to be a lifetime survival for a cancer patient who has successfully undergone treatment. The nurse I was speaking to told me how horrified she had been to learn this during her training. So did *my* lifespan now mean five years?

Realizing I still needed to learn a lot more, I found that the organization What Doctors Don't Tell You was holding a one-day conference on cancer in the centre of London. Tom and I attended and I felt further empowered when so many of my unspoken questions were being openly addressed by a team of highly regarded doctors from around the world. Refreshingly, nothing was being brushed aside; they had a different attitude to cancer and its treatment. Now I realized that it *was* possible for people to be successfully treated for cancer without intrusive, toxic chemotherapy.

4 Nursing the Wounds

October 2001

The appointment to find out from the haematology department why my body had lost so much blood and fluid in the operation brought no earth-shattering conclusion. It was decided that indeed, as I had suggested, my body had simply gone into shock and that it was 'just one of those things' ...

At the end of the third week of October, Tom came with me to an appointment for a prosthesis fitting. This took place in a small office-cum-stockroom in the basement in an old part of the Royal Marsden Hospital. On view were one or two bright, psychedelic-coloured wigs, the sort of thing you would normally choose for a Halloween night out – fun, providing you didn't have to wear it anywhere else. There were piles of boxes with different sized prostheses and, after being measured, I was offered a choice of two. Neither of them was a good fit, they were too big and to get the right size meant ordering and waiting a few weeks. We left without a satisfactory result. Later I went to a lingerie shop and got what I needed.

As no one seemed able to explain to me why I was having a problem with my eyelids not opening in the night, I made an appointment to see the eye specialist at the Royal Marsden. The appointment wasn't needed, for in the meantime Dr Rosy Daniel explained how chemotherapy could affect the eyes, and that she had come across this problem before. However, I now had another problem. My immediate concern was that after only two weeks I found my hair was beginning to fall out in large amounts. This was alarming and surprising when I remembered the woman patient who, after six chemotherapy treatments, had quite a reasonable amount of hair left. What was happening?

Losing my hair

My fears were soon realized. Despite only one shot of chemotherapy, because the nurse had been so uncertain about what to do with my hair and the ice cap, I might as well have gone without it for all the good it did. Quickly, over the next three weeks, my thick hair came out in huge chunks, particularly on the top of my head where the ice cap hadn't touched properly. This was the most enormous blow to me, and when I said how appalled I was during the haematology appointment, it was brushed aside with a cheerful 'Don't worry, it will come back thicker than before.' I found no comfort whatsoever in this reply. All along, the medical staff's cavalier approach, the 'arm's length' communication and flippant responses to my need for reassurance were staggering. To lose a breast was bad enough but to start losing all my hair now, when I'd had only one shot of chemotherapy, seemed a far worse blow than I could ever describe.

I recalled the heart-rending scenes of a World War II film showing French women labelled as traitors because they had harboured German soldiers. The women were subjected to a ritualized humiliation by having their heads shaved and being paraded through the streets for all to see. Now, just as I was regaining my intuition and instinct, I felt that I too was being subjected to some sort of punishment. The anger I felt was enormous. Was it purely a badly applied ice cap, or was it also something far worse, a possible overdose of chemotherapy? I will never know the truth, but it was devastating. It only served to confirm to me that my decision to quit was the best one to make.

Not only was my hair rapidly thinning, but I had to wear spectacles as the eye problem made it unwise to use contact lenses. It had taken only minutes – you might aptly say 'at the drop of a hat' – and I was looking pretty grim. Not easy for any middle-aged woman who is trying to make the best of herself; after all, these things are a huge part of our identity and I don't know what I would have done if I'd been due to give a concert at that time. Ask any woman what it feels like to watch her hair disappear and she will tell you, 'horrendous'. To have to carry off a Sinead O'Connor bald head at any age is cruel. The reality of it is as devastating as the breast operation, perhaps even more so as you can no longer conceal your illness from the world, just at a time when you need every resource possible to try to regain normality.

After only three weeks, Daphne came with me to find a wig which would look as much like my own hair as possible. The morning and afternoon's work resulted in the purchase of two pos-sibilities; meanwhile I rang my friend Gemma Herincx who makes wigs for the Royal Opera House, Covent Garden, for some advice. She immediately suggested that I spoke to her colleague Terri, who lived near to me, telling me that she would know how to make a wig look 'real'. Terri very generously arrived at my home a few days later, and when she saw the state of my own hair, agreed that I could be in for even further loss.

I begin to find those who offer wisdom

Around this time I decided to explore Neuro-Linguistic Programming (NLP), to provide me with a fast track in assisting the return of a healthy homeostasis. I had read a little about NLP, and remembered that my friend Nicci had spoken of an NLP course whilst Tom and I were in Spain for her wedding to Giulio. Maybe this could be a good idea for me too I promptly made enquiries and was put in touch with Medical NLP Master Practitioner Garner Thomson, who was to become hugely instrumental on my road to recovery.

By now my trust in the existing conventional system of treating breast cancer was about as low as it could be, and I felt the need to be in touch with other opinions. Then I remembered an old college friend, Sue Kümmel, who had married and gone to live in Germany. I hadn't spoken to her for a year or two, but remembered that she'd had breast cancer some years previously and was now completely recovered. So I telephoned her and filled her in on events to date, explaining how I felt the course of treatment being offered was too drastic. She suggested that I spoke with her friend Dr Angelika Vogel, a flautist in Sue's chamber music group in Germany. She gave me Angelika's telephone number and I arranged to talk to her the next evening. Speaking to Angelika was like a breath of fresh air. Her opinion was that radiotherapy was not the best option following mastectomy, and she told me that in Düsseldorf a very good breast clinic offered excellent advice. She also recommended that it could be worthwhile to enquire about some of the church-based clinics in the EU. Clearly there were other routes to be taken which were readily available and acknowledged in Germany unlike in the UK. She gave me lots of time to talk and suggested that I also spoke with her friend, the gynaecologist Dr Giesow, who had not recommended chemotherapy. Already I felt greatly uplifted, knowing that at last I had found a real empathy with my situation.

A day or two later I spoke with Dr Giesow and gained more excellent wisdom and information. Like Angelika, she asked for the background of events, telling me that natural science integrated with allopathic (conventional) medicine was a very good route and had produced extremely good results. It appears that, unlike in the UK, German private clinics offering this kind of approach were recognized by some German health insurance schemes. She gave me very useful guidance saying I should look to myself and see what I felt my needs were, and try to find a creative balance.

Statistics, she said, were uncertain, and definitions were vague and biased. Studies were a consensus which decides our corridor of knowledge – not what is true; neither did they take other factors into consideration. Here, at last, I knew I was speaking to a woman of integrity who was being true to her holistic beliefs, and was not prepared to accept the consensus view at face value. I felt in tune with all that she said. She suggested that I continue the helpful things I was already doing and strongly advised getting additional support from healing, which I was already doing, and told me that we had good Chinese medicine available in Buckinghamshire, although she didn't have the address. For further research, she recommended Professor Candace Pert, the American who discovered the brain's 'opiate receptor' in the 1970s. Later I was to learn of Professor Pert's involvement with NLP and it was becoming obvious that healthy coincidences were beginning to appear in my search.

Why couldn't I have had a conversation like this with the doctors who were looking after me while I followed the conventional treatment for breast cancer? Why is it that in some countries you might get your health insurers to cover you for other treatments that are not necessarily the standard cut, poison, burn (CPB) solution to breast cancer? Above all, how many more women like me are unaware of the successful breast cancer treatments available in other countries? At last, I was being informed of the sort of things that I needed to hear about, and every step began to reveal more.

My next trip to Breast Cancer Haven proved an eye-opener. I had arrived well before my appointment for cranial osteopathy with Chris, and decided to have lunch in the coffee shop. It was busy: the few tables were taken, so I joined two other women. On this unusually warm day, I was aware of two or three women wearing open neck blouses, revealing what looked like extensive burning. I was quietly horrified and later in conversation another woman declared that she would never let anyone see her chest as it was so badly damaged from radiation. Here in the closed environment of Breast Cancer Haven it was wonderful that these women could be together to bare and share, but how appalling to see these results of radiotherapy. Why? Was this unavoidable, or was it an act of carelessness in the administering of the treatment? Whatever the answer, I was extremely upset by what I was seeing and would need a great amount of convincing that radiation could ever be a safe choice for me.

Feeling empowered

It was this kind of encounter that fired my research – although it seemed like hacking into a deep, thorny forest, with no way of knowing if I could come out successfully intact, on the other side. Contradictions, bad choices disguised as good ones were now an everyday occurrence, but somehow I was becoming increasingly better at listening to my inner voice. I had to draw on all my own limited knowledge, rather like a new mother having to find a safe solution for a baby who is unwell. With all my instincts I *knew* that 'out there' was a superior solution and I needed to find it now for my own survival.

I remembered how my elder son at six years old had been suffering with a kind of allergic asthma, and how, after a chance encounter, I had first come across homeopathy. At the time I had been giving a concert for Sotheby's in Portsmouth and was staying with a professor of homeopathy and his wife in their magnificent house which Lord Nelson had bought for Lady Hamilton, so that she could wander through the beautiful garden, look directly out to sea and watch the fleet of ships passing to and fro. After the concert and a chance conversation over drinks, the professor's brother-in-law told me how he had been cured of asthma with homeopathy. Portsmouth was a long way from where we were living, so they suggested I enquire in the Harley Street area of London. There I found a homeopath and miraculously within six weeks my son was able to be free of almost 90 per cent of the allopathic medicine he had been taking.

Now, late in October, I thought that perhaps this could also help me, so I made an appointment with the same homeopathic practitioner. She asked me to bring all the information I had collected from the hospital, including the blood test results taken from the moment of diagnosis, plus a copy of the operation report. I didn't have this report, so I rang the doctor at the hospital day unit and requested a copy. After some difficulty I received it, and took it to my homeopathy appointment. I relayed my story, mentioning that three of the lymph nodes had been affected, and that I had decided I would not be having any more chemotherapy. She looked through the operation report, then suddenly, in an alarmed voice exclaimed, 'But it says here that you have six affected nodes!' I was shaken as I was hearing something now that I should have been told before I left hospital. What was going on? Why hadn't I been told? The hospital had not been honest with me and for what purpose? Were they trying to cover up the seriousness of the original, wrong diagnosis, thinking that it was better that I didn't know that things were even worse than I had already been told? The homeopath realized I was shocked, but my reaction was minor compared to hers. She hastily made a prescription and with great agitation told me that I should immediately go back to the hospital, as I might need more chemotherapy. I said nothing. I walked out of the practice on to the pavement and took a deep, calm breath. Boy oh boy! I really had landed in the jungle. This was the ultimate test. Which direction on this treacherous pathway should I take? I had now arrived at the point in the story when the transformation really took place; all that I'd done up to now, had empowered me, sustained me, and opened my eyes to see the truth.

Transformation

This time, I was definitely not prepared to think that a doctor knew better than I did. I would not be returning to the hospital for chemotherapy. More than that; actually there was no longer any need to panic: I had come such a long way by now and was learning all the time. So what! Three nodes or six – what was the difference? Resolutely, I refused to allow myself to be pulled down. I knew that I would never return to chemotherapy and that many people had fully recovered from far worse situations than mine without it. I also knew that after years of receiving homeopathic advice and treatment, I would not be returning to this particular surgery again. I needed people who were thinking and speaking the same language as me, who would be looking to a nurturing solution and be totally committed to help this miraculous thing called the body to heal itself. It would be pointless confronting anyone at the hospital about these new revelations, because I needed all my resources for keeping calm and creating my own good health. Neither would I tell Tom, for the time being, as I was not going to attach any importance to this latest development because there was nothing either of us could do about it anyway. What was the point of worrying? More bad news was a waste of his energy and mine. That was it then. I paused on the pavement, strangely content, and then moved on.

A joyful weekend

Happily, Saturday 29 October 2001 was a very significant day. Knowing I was not having any more chemotherapy, our dear friends Richard and Yvonne Sherrington had telephoned earlier in the week saying they would like to give a dinner party for me, thinking that it might give me a boost. Of course I was delighted. They gave me the choice of a quiet supper for the four of us, or a party of eight with mutual friends. Several of our friends were passionate about music including Richard, a benefactor of the ballet, and also founder of the Evening Standard Dance Awards, so this was a great lift to my spirit and I opted for a party of eight – the more the merrier! Dinner was organized to suit my organic diet, and everyone seemed to thoroughly relish the get-together; the whole evening was a joy. Richard insisted on playing my *Songs Without Words* album, so after dinner I suggested that we'd like to listen to something different, but he was having none of it. I was very touched by the generosity that both he and Yvonne had shown. They had been so supportive and concerned for me throughout my recovery, visiting me frequently. Somewhere around midnight we all departed, happy and relaxed. I felt that, at last, I had touched the life that I'd known before all the drama: a window of 'normality' had pleasantly opened up.

Improvisation – recording piano music without boundaries

After the weekend I had more cranial massage and acupuncture with Chris at Breast Cancer Haven, which I always found deeply relaxing. I was preparing in my mind the week ahead, and the planned recording session at home with Dave Lewis, my sound engineer. In furthering my efforts to come to a state of complete 'one-ness' in performance, I had decided to do a totally improvised recording. The whole idea of going into a studio, not knowing what I was going to play or how it would turn out, had a great appeal after a lifetime of daily practice and preparation of vast amounts of written works mainly for live performance. There were to be no boundaries, no margins and no place to go that could possibly be 'wrong', simply because there was no 'right' planned in the first place. I liked the idea, but also knew it was very much an experiment that might well land flat on its face. Although it didn't occur to me at the time, strangely, this seemed to coincide with my abandonment of the conventional medical treatment in order to find my own path: both were an experiment and a challenge, but not taken rashly.

Bad news

November 2001

The next day, I visited Garner Thomson for another excellent Medical NLP session from which I was now really beginning to feel some benefit. I was doing a twice daily 15-minute meditation specifically designed to evoke the healing response. None of this, however, could have prepared me for the evening telephone call from Yvonne to tell us that Richard had been killed in a car crash on the M25. Tom and I were devastated. I could not believe that Richard, who had shown such generosity of spirit and just helped me to joyfully regain some of my former self, was no longer with us. The wonderful dinner party had turned out to be his last. I had to decide whether or not to cancel my recording session the next day. Overwhelmed, for the first time I felt unable to face attending a funeral; it was this realization that gave me the incentive to do something positive. I would not be at the funeral, but I could go ahead with the recording session and dedicate it to Richard. I quickly decided that this was the best thing to do and rang Dave to warn him that the day might be a disaster – but what the hell – I'd give it my best shot because it seemed the only way to say 'Thank you' to Richard.

The next morning I lit a candle for Richard, then Dave and I quietly set up to record. We began the session on the understanding that every take was to be kept, regardless of mistakes, unless they were clearly unusable. It turned out to be an amazing day. The music seemed to unfold in its own way without any pressure, and both Dave and I knew that all the recordings could be used. There was more to do, but it was a very promising start. In the evening I phoned Yvonne and told her that I intended to dedicate the music to Richard, as it seemed the best that I could do for both of them. She was very touched and comforted at the idea.

Picking up the pieces

Over the next few days, life continued as normally as possible, in the circumstances. Another vitamin C infusion and, at my ever-encouraging friend Anton Mullan's instigation, a visit to the BBC with a view to them using some of my music, although my main preoccupation was to get back to full health again. Two days later I had an appointment at the Royal Marsden with the doctor in charge of radiotherapy. By now I had done enough research to know that it was extremely unlikely that I would take the treatment. At my appointment I listened to figures which indicated that I would be better off doing it, and then I asked the questions about the possible side effects. I was concerned that my heart could be affected by the radiotherapy treatment to the left side of my chest. The reply was that it was possible. What about my work as a musician, using fingers, hands and arms continually – would there be more likelihood of lymphodoema in the arm? 'Yes, that is possible.' Had women become completely free from cancer without radiotherapy? 'Yes, they had.' These were just a few of the questions and replies. The doctor felt that I wasn't ready to receive radiotherapy and I told her that I really didn't think I wanted it. She suggested I call her office, having had time to think about it, and said she was interested that I was using nutrition to help myself, adding that she wanted to know more about the effects of diet in breast cancer.

During the same week I had what was to be my last attempt at giving conventional UK cancer treatment a hearing. Dr Denning suggested that I made a private appointment at the Cromwell Hospital with Professor Michael Baum, an expert in the field of breast cancer. I was glad to have his second opinion, but found that the figures he gave for the success rates of chemotherapy were not as high as had been previously indicated to me, and there was the added problem of being thrown into the menopause rather abruptly, particularly around the age of 50. I voiced my belief that the arrival of my lump, so soon after having a mammogram, was not a coincidence and found a receptive ear to my growing distrust in the safety of mammograms. However, Professor Baum said he supported the idea of radiotherapy and regarded it as important to take tamoxifen for five years. (About this time there was news on television and in the newspapers that treatment with tamoxifen for five years was too long and it was to be cut to about two and a half years). He was extremely excited about a new preparation currently on trial called Arimidex, which he believed was a major break-through and would be very effective, saying it was likely to be available shortly, even in the next month or so. Later, I discovered that some of these new drugs, unlike tamoxifen, actually shut down the body's oestrogen supply altogether and that women need the 'good' oestrogen produced in the body. So why annihilate it all? I have since found other doctors who shared my scepticism of these new drugs. More and more, I was seeing division amongst the medical profession as to which was the best way to treat breast cancer.

There also seemed to be varying attitudes to the types of tamoxifen available. I was troubled with digestive problems, one of the several side effects of tamoxifen. After discussing this with the surgeon, Mr Sacks, he prescribed a different type from the one I had been using. A week or two later, when the prescription had not arrived, I rang the hospital pharmacy to be told that they did not know of this particular, prescribed variety of the drug, and anyway, their policy was to issue whatever type of tamoxifen the pharmaceutical companies sent them.

Time for contemplation

December 2001

I had an increasing sense of wanting to be on my own, with time to reflect and take stock of my situation. I continued to understand more about my dietary needs, regularly practised Tai Chi, took supplements and vitamin C infusions and meditated daily. In addition, I had regular acupuncture sessions with Ana Maria Lavin Parot at The Kailash Centre in St John's Wood and gradually began to feel stronger, but it was becoming clear to me that I must find a new perspective on my situation. Tom was working full-time at home, finishing his book, *The Boiled Frog Syndrome*, about health and the built environment. Consequently our life revolved entirely around the home and, although Tom helped tremendously with everything, my days seemed completely bound up with domesticity, mostly in the kitchen juicing and making organic meals. I continued to see a few students, which always gave me a great lift. Nevertheless, something needed to change. Should I go away and take a cottage somewhere to provide me with the solitude that I was seeking? It was winter and not the best time to be away. I felt unsettled.

One December morning, during a meditation, a strange thing happened. As I was well into the meditation and feeling in a deep, calm place, a picture framed in a small circle emerged in front of my closed eyes. In the middle of the circle was a pair of climbing boots and it was almost like seeing them in a hologram. They were so vivid and real that, although still in meditation, I felt a strong urge to put my hand out to touch them. Of course I couldn't as my body was inert, just as it would be when asleep at night and dreaming. I had never experienced anything so 'real' in a meditation before, and it was something that I was certainly not going to forget, despite there seeming to be no relevance whatsoever in the climbing boots. Although I did possess a pair of climbing boots and always enjoyed walking, I had not used them since my visit to the foothills of the Himalayas some six years before. I put the incident to the back of my mind and carried on with the daily meditations. It was going to be Christmas before long, and I reckoned it would be great to be at home with the family, especially as I was in such good practice domestically and, best of all, I was still here.

5 A New Pathway

Tom and I ended 2001 in Brighton, taking our first weekend away since my breast cancer diagnosis. The hotel served organic food, our room overlooked the sea and it was a luxury not to be cooking. The sea air gave us a well-needed lift to end the year.

January arrived. What was I going to do now that I had abandoned the conventional treatment for breast cancer? Some of the places offering alternative treatment that Tom and I had looked into were interesting, but not thoroughly convincing and quite expensive. We discussed this at some length, and agreed that I should talk to Dr Rosy Daniel. I asked Rosy what she'd do if she was in my situation, and after some thought she came up with a couple of suggestions, adding that she would be inclined to see someone like Dr Fritz Schellander at the Liongate Clinic in Tunbridge Wells. I made an appointment to see him on 16 January. Meanwhile I visited Vanessa Bailey, the trichologist at John Bell and Croyden, the chemists in Wigmore Street, who gave me constructive help with my hair which was still falling out. It was reassuring to talk to someone who understood the problem and her examination showed that despite the devastation created by the chemotherapy there was good reason to hope that my hair would return, but it would take time. Meanwhile my research continued, and the pile of copious notes steadily grew as friends sent me information about women who had been successfully treated for breast cancer by other methods.

As I walked up the hill to my appointment with Dr Schellander, legs still pacing themselves steadily as energy seemed low, I paused for a break outside a jeweller's shop. There in the window was a delicate pair of earrings similar to some which I had seen in London, but here they were very reasonably priced and on the spur of the moment I went in and bought them. Delighted, the rest of the uphill journey felt much lighter and the earrings became a talisman for my solidarity in the task of regaining my wholeness and health: a symbol of the hope of good things to come, along with a beautiful gold ring which Tom had given me for Christmas. A sort of completion.

A new, refreshing outlook

I arrived at the Liongate Clinic and was shown into the waiting room. On the table were files of success stories of patients who had been given chelation therapy treatment in Dr Schellander's clinic. Until then I knew very little about chelation, so this was particularly interesting as I recalled that it was a therapy suggested by Dr Lorraine Day in her inspiring cancer video. Essentially, it appears that the treatment is for patients with heart problems and chelation is administered through a drip, so it is very similar to receiving a vitamin infusion. It removes toxins and the arteries are cleared out, frequently saving patients from risky, intrusive heart surgery. After taking chelation, many of these patients can do things they were unable to do before – free of pain. In some cases they are able to take up quite strenuous sports which previously would have been impossible. I found Dr Schellander's thoughtful approach unhurried and refreshing. He wanted to know everything: my background, my children, my work, my parents, and how they had died. Then he explained how the body is very often depleted of adrenaline when cancer occurs. This was news to me and made complete sense. He had astutely observed that I was the type of person who felt a need to put a great energy into what I was doing, often stretching beyond the norm in order to do so. This was true as I had tried, following my mother's illness and death, to make sure I did everything possible to make my life meaningful and successful. I had had a similar attitude after my divorce, becoming the breadwinner, bringing up my sons and creating a successful career. Now suddenly, for the first time, pieces of my life's jigsaw were coming together. I remembered performing in *What's the Score?* the previous April and not being able to understand the lack of an adrenaline rush. I immediately told Dr Schellander about this experience as I was certain my adrenaline had not been functioning properly. Everything he was saying was making sense. For the first time I was excited, knowing that I was close to discovering something exceedingly important and I needed to know more.

A gut feeling I must pursue

Dr Schellander told me that a colleague and friend of his in Germany had discovered a way of successfully treating cancer – even in patients with quite advanced tumours – by restoring their adrenaline system and returning them to full health, without any recurrence. Her name was Dr Waltraut Fryda. Now in her seventies, she had been working with cancer patients for over forty years at her practice near the mountains of southern Bavaria. Instantly, the shelved memory of the climbing boots from my meditation flashed before my eyes. It was an extraordinary moment, suddenly everything was falling into place and whatever I had been waiting for had arrived. How should I contact her? What should I do next? Dr Schellander gave me her phone number and suggested the best time to talk to her. I left, feeling that whatever the outcome I must go to Bavaria to meet her.

February 2002

The next day I called Germany and spoke with Dr Fryda's assistant and then with Dr Fryda herself. She sounded good, no frills or lengthy explanations and said that she would see me. That weekend I prepared for the trip, packing an overnight bag and taking an overcoat in case it was cold. I planned to fly to Munich on Tuesday 4 February, hire a car and be at her surgery the following morning.

Sitting on the plane I recalled my telephone conversation with Dr Fryda and the information about her treatment from Dr Schellander. In my mind's eye I had created a vision of what the place I was going to would look like: it gave me a very good feeling. I picked up the car at Munich airport and began my journey south. As I finally left the autobahn, which continued on to Salzburg, I began travelling across a very peaceful and beautiful landscape. The air felt amazingly fresh after London as I drove through large expanses of green and open farmland dotted with typical Bavarian houses and farms: above me – a huge wash of blue sky. Finally I arrived at the small hamlet of Kreuth and my hotel. The area gently nestled in a valley under the gaze of the huge mountain, Wallberg, a part of the Alps. The contrast with the frantic pace and pollution of London could not have been greater. Here was complete tranquillity connected to a different kind of reality, one which respected the natural world and its rhythms. It seemed to represent a symbolic healing journey: it was the soul of the territory of my 'vision' of the climbing boots. Here was enormous peace.

The following morning, I arrived at Dr Fryda's surgery and was shown into the calm and well cared for waiting room with comfortable seats and a table full of magazines. Leaflets and other information were placed to one side of the room and beautiful plants in the window opposite. It was not large, but had a light, airy feel about it; quite unlike many impersonal, utilitarian surgeries. I had not been waiting for many minutes when I heard a voice greet me: 'Mrs Saunders, hello, I am Dr Fryda.' There stood a tall, very elegant woman with dark hair – although I knew that she was over 70 – looking much younger than she really was. She shook my hand and invited me into her surgery. I sat in front of her large desk, my eyes resting on a stunning, bright pink azalea. This was different to any doctor's surgery that I had been in before. I can only describe the feeling as one of total warmth and welcome: that certainly was something new.

Out of the forest and into the clearing

I realized within a few moments that I was talking to a woman of tremendous depth and understanding, not just about my illness but concerning people and what makes them tick. It soon became clear how Dr Fryda regarded all the aspects – psychological, mental, emotional and spiritual – as fundamental to the whole person, whether they were well or ill. The wonderful and rather unusual thing was that at the same time, she was a scientist. To find a combination of the two in such magnitude and balance seemed remarkable, especially since I had spent so much time already with doctors supposedly knowledgeable in the field of cancer, who appeared to regard the patient like a machine that had gone wrong, with their job being to fix it. I had problems with this attitude. It simply didn't fit in to my understanding of the awesome complexity of human beings and our universe. I soon learned that in her long career Dr Fryda had spent many years in research in order to understand the journey of cancer from its outset to the arrival of the tumour. I knew I was going to learn much more, but for now she had a string of questions to ask me, not only about the blood tests which I had brought along, but also the pattern of my life up to now. 'What happened to you about fifteen years ago?' she asked. A quick reckoning took me back to the end of my divorce. 'That,' she said, 'is significant in your illness, and cancer is an illness and should be treated as such.' She went on to tell me how cancer can start in the body many years before the symptoms appear and how the body needs rest and care when we are ill, which in the modern world we tend to overlook by continuing to work 'through it', often to our later cost. The lack of adrenaline impairs the immune system and causes other problems, making the body 'available' to cancer. She had found that cancer patients were often very low in adrenaline, sometimes not even registering any at all. Although my adrenaline had never been tested, I told her how I instinctively felt that it was low. She outlined a course of treatment which meant that I would have to live nearby for seven weeks, seeing her daily at the surgery to receive injections to regenerate my system, to monitor my progress and, she hoped, to turn around the illness to get rid of any possible cancer. She suggested that I might like to go back to London, give it some thought and call her later. If I wanted to start the treatment, then it could be arranged quite soon.

A very special doctor

Without hesitation I told her that I wanted to start immediately. There was no point in going back to London when I could begin to get well straight away. I only had an overnight bag with me, but knew I wouldn't need much and Tom could probably bring me a suitcase with everything I might need for the seven weeks. She laughed, and seeing that I was in no doubt, gave me the address of the nearby information centre where they would help me find a bedsit with a kitchen, as I was to be doing my own cooking according to her special diet.

As soon as I left the surgery I called Tom. He thought it was a great idea to stay and said he would book a flight for the weekend – only a few days away. Off I went to the information centre to find a long list of holiday letting accommodation, many houses having small apartments as the area is very popular for skiing and walking. By the end of the afternoon I had made arrangements to stay in a bedsit belonging to Frau Franck and her husband Reinhard, both professional musicians which seemed a good omen. My room was at the top of the house, decorated and furnished throughout with pine. It was modern and neat with a double bed on one side and on the other, in a corner, seating built around a dining table, where I could read, write and watch television. The double French windows opened onto a tiny balcony looking out across the mountains – a great bonus and a good way to test the outside temperature. Off the main room, a skylight brightened the well kitted out galley kitchen and at the far end there was a very small but adequate bathroom with a shower. No luxuriating in a bath for a few weeks, but so what? This was all mine – along with the peace that I had been searching for: I could not have wished for more. I postponed my return flight and extended my car hire at a very reasonable rate.

The next morning I attended the surgery and was greeted with a very cheerful 'Good morning' from a young woman with an Irish accent. Up to now, everyone that I had spoken to had been German, so it came as a surprise. Her name was Irene Henchy, a tall vivacious blonde, who had come from Ireland the previous week with her husband and two young sons to begin her treatment for breast cancer. We arranged to meet later at the local café, along with her husband Michael and younger son, four-year-old Joey (think more *Sound of Music* than Hard Rock Café, with Tyrolean-style trimmed tablecloths). The café's speciality was *Sachertorte*, an exceptionally smooth, rich chocolate cake originally from the Hotel Sacher in Vienna. Because of Dr Fryda's diet the cake was now forbidden to me and Irene, but a treat for Michael and Joey. We poured out our stories to each other. Irene had undergone surgery in Ireland, a month or two previously, for a lumpectomy and removal of the lymph nodes. She had been told by the doctors to have a mastectomy and removal of the lymph glands a couple of weeks later. Irene refused to do this, in spite of being told that there were also two tumours on her lymph nodes and very possibly more affected. It had been a battle, but she stood her ground despite her doctor getting very angry about her refusal to undergo chemo-therapy and radiotherapy. Her husband Michael had stepped in, telling the doctor that she felt very emotional about everything and although she was not saying a definite 'no' to further treatments, she needed time to consider carefully. The doctor told him that he could give her pills for the emotional problem so as not to lose time. Irene felt unhappy about the prospect of chemotherapy, par-ticularly as she did not feel ill. She had left hospital the day after the lumpectomy and couldn't come to terms with having to become sick by taking chemotherapy when she felt so well, knowing it gave no guarantee of a cure. Finally, she decided that this sort of treatment was 'out' as far as she was concerned. Her reasons were straightforward, she wanted some quality of life, to be able to pick up her child, and the risk of lymphodoema was something she was not prepared to tolerate, along with the possibility of an early menopause due to breast cancer drugs. Irene had visited what she described as a 'wise woman' at home in Ireland. The woman had helped many people with advice about natural and alternative treatment and, thinking that it would be important for Irene to boost her system in readiness should she decide to go ahead with the hospital treatment, she had suggested that Irene visit Dr Schellander in Tunbridge Wells as part of the process. Irene came to England and took Dr Schellander's chelation therapy treatment for a week and was told of Dr Fryda's treatment, which she reckoned sounded a far better solution than the treatment she had been offered in Ireland. I was tremendously impressed by her positive attitude and determination to follow her path with Dr Fryda and it was a good feeling to know that I was not alone.

By the end of our exchanges and several cups of tea later, the other customers had left and the café looked deserted. Suddenly, Michael, in his southern Irish lilt burst out – 'I don't believe it! Oh my! Joey…!' Irene joined in – as we turned to see that young Joey had been keeping himself occupied throughout by carefully removing the sugar bowls from each table and neatly lining them up on the large table in the front window, giving the appearance of 15 or so sparkling-white sugar mountains. A four-year-old's homage to the Alps perhaps? It certainly looked like it. Clearly there were more pressing matters than our breast cancer: life had to go on – thank God there was a parallel universe to ours – Joey's.

Tom arrived at the weekend with a large suitcase. I didn't require lots of clothing, simply things to keep me warm and comfortable for the inevitable snow, plus a pair of high heels and one reasonably smart suit, just in case I needed them. The magic climbing boots were essential for the walks in all kinds of weather and so they finally came out again for the first time since their last sojourn in India. There were kitchen utensils, CDs, books, including a couple of 'teach yourself German' books – my knowledge of the language being very limited – and finally, sheet music and music-manuscript paper. The likelihood of my using the manuscript paper was not great; somehow in my heart it didn't seem the right time for being highly creative in anything, other than getting well. It was time now to take stock and see things anew. During the weekend Tom and I shared a little of the magic of Bavaria and, although I needed to be on my own, I knew I would miss him terribly and have to wait until his next visit in a week or two. On Sunday, I drove him to Munich airport, feeling sad to see him go and saving the tears for after he had disappeared. Now I had to get into the rhythm of living another life and experience the unknown for a while, safe and firm in the belief that I had made the right choice for myself.

Dr Fryda took blood tests, which were to be repeated regularly throughout the treatment. The tests covered all the standard requirements of those done at the Royal Marsden, but included many more with some covering the status of vitamins, minerals and hormones in detail. A urine test was taken to check the level of adrenaline. I had with me the previous results from the Royal Marsden which included cancer markers. She warned me that over the next weeks it was quite possible that the cancer markers would rise and then they would drop, probably quite dramatically! I had no difficulty in believing her as her track record in itself was enough to convince me, plus the fact that the tests were soon to prove, just as I'd thought, that my adrenaline was so low that it wasn't registering at all. My experience of conventional breast cancer treatment had given me the impression that thyroid function is often disregarded, or considered unimportant. The new tests showed that mine was low, as were the results for some other functions. Dr Fryda was quick to begin correcting all these, for she viewed them as an essential part of the rebalancing on the journey back to health. I was given the necessary medication to correct my thyroid levels plus vitamin and mineral supplements. This only served to support all that I had first suspected about my illness; the realization that several things were out of balance and how that *must* affect the rest of the body, further convincing me that this was exactly the treatment that I should be having. The only thing left of my treatment in London was the tamoxifen. I hadn't stopped taking it as I was so sure I must reduce my oestrogen levels, so what, I wondered, was her view on this. She made it clear that it was no big issue. I could carry on taking it if it made me feel more secure, but it was not vital to her course of treatment. By choice, some patients continued long after the treatment was ended, whilst others never took it at all. I continued for a few months, reducing it gradually and making a total of nine to ten months of taking it. I signed a form confirming that I had refused the further treatment I had been offered in the UK, including chemotherapy.

A joint commitment to regain my health

The whole treatment was to take two years, the first year to be based on whatever treatment Dr Fryda thought appropriate as a result of the seven-week stay. For the second year I simply had to keep to the diet and any supplements that might be required. I was to be in bed around 10pm each night for a long time ahead, not get overstressed about anything and have good regular exercise, which meant a daily one-hour walk, unless for any reason I felt unduly tired. Clearly I was to play a vital part in my own healing, and walking in this idyllic countryside was going to be rather like being on a glorious holiday.

At long last my diet, crucial to the healing process, was under medical supervision, while going shopping each day for fresh food was a luxury that I would not have had time for at home. The local supermarkets and the *Markthalle* provided me with fresh organic fruit and vegetables and the butcher also sold fresh fish. The main 'bio' shop (the German equivalent of our organic shop) had bread, sugar-free jams, dairy (not too high a fat content) and soya produce plus the occasional treat of a snack bar made with honey. Sugar was banned, but some honey and fructose were allowed. Bananas – very high in sugar – grapes, sultanas, currants and peanuts were forbidden; however, dried apricots became a good substitute, especially for baking. Everything had to be wholegrain and organic including bread, pasta and rice; both fresh and dried herbs could be used and some frozen vegetables were allowed in small amounts. Nothing refined or processed and nothing in a tin or preserved: malt extracts, saccharin and additives were out! Olive oil and cooking oils needed to be cold pressed, good quality and if I felt like baking a cake there was no problem, as I could sweeten it with honey or fructose and use a special type 1050 wholewheat flour – so much finer than the rather heavy wholewheat baking flour I had tried using at home. A drink of wine with supper was a surprise perk and something to look forward to occasionally; likewise the one or two cups of high-quality coffee each day which Dr Fryda did not see as a problem, along with herbal and green teas and the fresh or unsweetened fruit juices which I enjoyed. Drinking the local tap water was an unexpected bonus as it was crystal clear from the mountains, saving me from having to buy bottled water. As far as meat was concerned, pork, sausages, smoked and preserved meats were banned, but some organic meat such as lamb, chicken, turkey, other poultry and beef were fine. During the initial seven weeks only fish was allowed, as long as it wasn't smoked – no meat until the treatment was complete.

Dealing with nagging fears

My days soon settled into a kind of routine. From Monday to Friday after breakfast I would go to the surgery, arriving between nine and ten. Each day Dr Fryda would be ready to discuss anything I might want to ask her. I would then receive injections which were to encourage the body to regenerate its own healing. The regeneration injections are German products and they are not 'alternative' but allopathic medicine. Dr Fryda has a vast knowledge of their detailed properties and is able to tailor a therapy to the individual's needs. The procedure was simple, quick and painless. On one of the morning visits to the surgery, Dr Fryda was asking questions about my general health and if there was anything troubling me that I hadn't mentioned as it was vital that she knew. Although it didn't seem that significant, I told her of a slightly nagging cough, which I reckoned (and hoped) was due to a sinus 'drip' made worse in the morning after lying down all night. She immediately ordered a chest X-ray, and told me that I must drive to a clinic in Bad Tolz, as this was the best place to have it taken. Things were moving quickly, with everything being thoroughly checked and no delays in making appointments.

Bad Tolz is a pretty place, the town divided by a bridge over the beautiful river Isar and the clinic not far from the town centre. The interior of the clinic was fresh and modern and I had been in the reception area only three or four minutes when a woman radiographer arrived, took me to a changing room and asked me to strip to the waist, saying that she would be back shortly. I stood in front of the mirror as I took my bra off and felt uncomfortable and embarrassed about my mastectomy. Of course it was no problem to the medical staff and my 'bad' moment was quickly over when I began the X-rays.

The machinery seemed very modern and sparkling compared to that at home. I didn't have long to wait and was told that the doctor would be in to see me shortly. No sooner had she spoken than in walked the doctor of every woman's dreams: tall, tanned, handsome and I'd say around fifty. He was absolutely gorgeous. In a gentle voice and speaking perfect English, he told me he wanted to take some more X-rays, which were done on a machine unlike anything I had seen before, giving what seemed to be a 360° picture of my lungs. After a few minutes he said, 'I'm pleased to tell you that everything is normal.' My relief was enormous. The most likely cause was, as I had suspected, the sinuses – made worse with the winter.

I dressed and sat in reception in order to pay my bill – much less expensive than in London and with the added benefit of excellent equipment, not to mention an exceptional doctor! After waiting some minutes, to my surprise he came out to see me again, although we had said goodbye. He sat down beside me and asked if I had considered a reconstruction. I immediately told him how bad I felt about not having a breast and yes, I'd thought about it quite a lot, but for the future when I knew the time was right. He told me of a plastic surgeon he had recently visited in Munich, whose work he considered to be of a particularly high standard and gave me the surgeon's card. His thoughtfulness, concern and again the time given to talk was wonderful and I left feeling much lighter than before. 'Much lighter' is probably an understatement as I headed for a most beautiful church nearby and sat alone, so incredibly grateful for all that I had, for my family and all the care that I was being given. I had nothing more than breast cancer and I felt I was going to recover.

As I reflected on all that had happened, it seemed amazing how this whole journey had gathered momentum since Dr Rosy Daniel had set the ball rolling. From the minute I landed in Germany, all my worries were being taken care of so efficiently.

6 A Healing Refuge

Thursday 21 February 2002

It's nearly three weeks now since I arrived, and today is quite surreal. The mountains are enveloped in a snow-falling greyness. The Olympics at Salt Lake City are not having as much snow as this right now.

My room glows a stark white from the big window and the snow-covered skylight makes the place darker. I haven't had to drive in such conditions for years and it feels strangely pleasant. The roads are cleared very promptly – not easy with the amount of snow that continues to fall today. Back indoors it's a relief to take my wig off, although it certainly helps to keep my head warm, and at night I keep a woolly hat beside the bed in case it gets chilly. My hair is ridiculously thin and what's left is looking very grey at the front. I've just opened my door to find Frau Franck on her knees, cleaning the stairs. What a disaster! I've forgotten to put my wig on, so within a moment of her looking up I make a swift reappearance – 'transformed' after grabbing my blonde wig and tying the hair back in an extremely luxuriant version of the grey hair she has momentarily clapped her eyes on. She will either believe that she has a mad woman staying in her very pleasant accommodation, or hopefully, she might think that she was seeing things, and that the flash of a grey head was a momentary aberration on her part – the result of cleaning two flights of stairs a little too zealously!

I console myself with the fact that looking up from her kneeling position, she couldn't see the bald patch on top and that with luck my reappearance was merely an adjustment of the 'colour setting' in her mind. Let's face it, I really wanted everyone to believe that the wig was my own hair and I've just blown my cover. Ah, well – you can't win them all!

I've done the main shop of the week, mostly bio fresh fruit and vegetables, at the *Markthalle*. The owner came to chat to me – she speaks good English – and commented on the fact that I obviously liked to cook. Truth is, I'm enjoying cooking for myself, which is surprising even to me: life is so basic and earthy at the moment that my self-nurturing feels just right. Every evening I massage my head with the hair stimulant drops from Vanessa, hoping to help the regrowth. Tonight, both the Francks are playing in a sextet in Munich – rather them than me in this weather.

Friday 22 February

This morning, after visiting the surgery and breakfast, armed with a pile of piano music borrowed from Dr Fryda, I drove to the *Kuramt* (the local information hall) to play sonatinas and impromptus by Clementi, Schubert and Mozart for a couple of hours. It feels strange, almost eerie, playing this great German music so close to where it was written.

The Winter Olympics on television are great, especially when you are watching in a place similarly covered in snow. The British (Scots) girls are amazing at curling, their skipper a real warrior, honing all their skills to the ultimate and winning gold medals – the best in the whole tournament!

I visited Thomas who runs *Wallberg-Apotheke*, the chemist shop, in the hope of getting the English translation to the last of the injections which I needed to forward to the UK. Although he tried, the company involved seemed to be offhand about sending the information. I can only keep calling in to see if there's any joy. The receptionist to plastic surgeon Dr Gabka in Munich appeared to be equally offhand or was simply having a 'bad hair day' – which I understand only too well! Dr Fryda stepped in, pulling rank and putting her in her place by telling her we did not want 'enquiries' and that I needed to see Dr Gabka as soon as possible. Nice one. The next day a fax arrived offering an appointment. When I rang back, the receptionist greeted me quite delightfully – bad hair day presumably over!

It is 4.35pm, looking greyer than ever with plenty of snow falling. I wonder how it will be with Dr Gabka. It's a plan for the future, even a year or so away, but it will be good to know whether or not he can do a simple breast reconstruction or if the small amount of flesh I appear to have left is going to make it more complicated Who knows? Fortunately there are only two mirrors in this place so I'm not frequently confronted with my reflection. A lack of self-criticism is healthy right now – I don't need to be doing a heavy number on myself. In fact it seems, long term, a few 'reconstructions' would be a good idea and a 'lift' here and a tuck there would be rather welcome. This is a little surprising as I'd always believed I would be content to let the ageing process unfold naturally. There is nothing 'natural' about losing a breast and I seem to be forced down an avenue that I never envisaged. Before the mastectomy I had a quite reasonable pair of tits, now I have to find a way to make the best of a bad job so to speak. In addition, a part of me wants vindication which goes something like this: 'If modern surgery can be so sweeping and brutal in its approach to breast cancer – especially with a mastectomy – then it can also set to work to compensate and reinstate something of me that's been taken and whilst they're at it tweak a few other things into shape!' Well, I'll have to wait and see what *may* be possible. Irene has offered to come with me to Munich to see Dr Gabka: it will be an interesting day out next week.

Saturday 23 February

A great day in Innsbruck – a very pretty town surrounded by mountains and an atmosphere of winter sports. Irene and I have decided to return here in two years' time, to visit the *Sachertorte*

Café where we can indulge as a celebration. Whilst we were having lunch Tom phoned to say he was coming on Friday: a wonderful surprise – it will be *so* good to have him here again.

Sunday 24 February

The Salt Lake Olympics are awesome, but I see time slipping by quickly. It is crazy to think that there are still not enough hours in the day.

One of the best things that has happened is that my musical 'perfect' pitch which seemed to have dropped down a half tone, is mysteriously back on target again. With an 'A' tuning fork I can test it and every time it's coming up spot on. Strange, but I've just remembered that the last time I was aware of my pitch 'slipping' was years ago when I was going through a difficult patch. Who said illness is all physical? It just can't be true. I wish my German speaking was progressing just as well, it really needs regular, daily work and I'm desperate not to regiment my days, as they're already structured around visits to the doctor and cooking.

My God! Maggie Smith and Bette Midler are on television dubbed in German. Weird. Especially Maggie's distinctive voice – now completely lost. Is anyone in Germany aware of this? They'd certainly get a shock if they heard her true voice – not to mention the shock Maggie would get if she heard this – it's quite hilarious!

Monday 25 February

Two days of wild weather and today it has rained like there's no tomorrow. Even so, the snow is still everywhere. I am reading about the voice movement therapy by Paul Newham which is very heavy reading but compelling all the same. Tom will be here on Friday – can't wait.

Tuesday 26 February

Irene and I circumnavigated the southern side of the Munich ring road – not easy – but managed to jump off at the appropriate exit, more by good luck than anything else. In a tree-lined street we found Dr Gabka's smart, ultramodern clinic inside a grand, beautiful house. He soon appeared, energetic and smiling and looked to be about 40. First I introduced myself and then Irene, explaining who she was. I watched him turn towards her, quickly eyeing her up and down. 'Excellent,' I thought, 'he clearly loves women,' vital, as far as I was concerned, if his surgery for reconstruction was to be as good as I'd been told.

In his bright and airy room he sat facing me and examined my scar. I felt very comfortable speaking with him and he told me that in Germany they did not cut a mastectomy in the same way as in the UK, preferring to use an angle which would better conceal in a later reconstruction; however he could do a reconstruction that would look wonderful and he explained the options. The two best possibilities seemed to be either a body fat replacement taken from the tummy which is a much longer operation, or the least invasive method using a silicone implant. For either procedure, three pints of my blood would be needed beforehand. This precaution seemed to be a great idea, especially as I had lost a lot of blood during the mastectomy and didn't want a repeat of that. As part of the procedure they would run a routine test for cancer on the existing breast. He showed me lots of pictures of his reconstruction work and later I was able to see more of them on his website. It all looked promising. He gave me time to talk things through and left me in no doubt that although I knew it would not be for quite some time – at least a year or two – when I felt ready, he'd be able to do a marvellous job.

Lifted in spirits, Irene and I went into the centre of Munich for a late lunch, picking our way carefully through the menu to find suitable food. As we were eating, Irene caught sight of a woman with a plate of scones and cream. 'Oh, just look at that!' she drooled. It set me thinking – I had an idea. It seemed to me that many standard recipes could be adapted to our diet with just a little imagination. This was to be the start of a liberating collection of recipes and cooking experiments.

Thursday 7 March

Yesterday and today I've felt sluggish, despite trying to shake it off with a walk along the riverside to Kreuth and back. Whilst I'm here I must really set my sights: it's time to go out on a limb, some new inner move. I can sense where I'm looking, but now I have to take action. Perhaps this is an inner clock preparing me for my return home. Once I return, I know there will be a lot of support and the day-to-day routine of the last five weeks has shown me a new way of being. Nothing feels rushed here and I've found a wholeness which has brought me clarity. I look to the future with a better understanding of what I want and need. When I return home to London, I must act on it to secure the new path.

Reading back in 2006 through these diary entries, I recall that it was at about this point in my journey that I had discovered Joni Mitchell's album *From Both Sides Now* and fallen totally in love with it. Her voice sits in a simple, truthful and flowing place as she reclaims lyrics of other writers as if they were her own. As a musician, one area integral to my everyday work, that never ceases to fascinate me, is that of musical arranging. Here, on Joni's album, the score is lavishly arranged and performed by the best, including Wayne Shorter, Herbie Hancock and a huge orchestral line-up. I have always regarded writing a melodic line as the relatively easy part of composing; what really matters is the way the rhythms, harmonies, orchestration, spacing and colours of sound serve to create the perfect integration into the words and emotion of the songs. For me, this album comes as close to fulfilling this as any could. Here is a hero's journey through love, from the first moment of infatuation to the end of the affair and the philosophical understanding that something has been learned. Over the weeks I thrived on these songs as I walked along the wooded footpath by the river surrounded with the peacefulness and towering beauty of the mountains. Often, for instinctive self-preservation at this time, I would fast-forward the sad songs of a broken love affair to something more uplifting or philosophical. Even the first song, heralding the initial attraction, I would sometimes skip and go to the second track – *At Last* – a 1940s song by Harry Warren and Mack Gordon. This track, a total rejoicing and celebration of finding true love, was my favourite and my inspiration, followed closely by Joni's own song *From Both Sides Now*. All this helped me to put a perspective on my existence and somehow added to the positive health creation that I was experiencing. However, as a bonus, *At Last … My love has come along,* served as an anticipation of Tom's visits to me. Because I was so separated from him in distance, his visits became like a new love affair, as I waited eagerly for his arrival at the airport. To be able to show him my discovery of another beautiful view, order our food in my 'best' German, or take him by cable car to the top of a mountain, was all a contribution to our tender and precious time together before I would return him to the airport and say goodbye for another week or two.

Friday 8 March
Blood tests. As Dr Fryda expected, one marker raised and my white cells down a bit. Perhaps this is why I feel sluggish. Off now to Munich airport to meet Tom – it feels like an age since we've been together and I miss him badly.

Monday 11 March
A heavenly weekend. Seeing Tom off yesterday evening was hard. For the first time I wanted to go back home with him. We visited Tegernsee, the most beautiful lake and not far from here. From the nearby small town of Rottach-Egern the road winds around the large lake, the far end going on towards Munich. Tegernsee itself is a string of well-kept hotels, small shops and restaurants bordering the right-hand side of the lake, with its own prettily laid out flower beds appearing from time to time beside the attractive Bavarian houses as the road twists and bends. Apparently, the lake can often be frozen over in the winter, but as the warmer weather appears, so do the boats and many people come to swim. A regular ferry goes across and around, dropping off at other small, equally delightful places. Even in the cool, Tom and I were able to sit beside the lake

and enjoy the warmth of the sun, later watching it drop down, golden, over the water. I took him to Bad Wiesse, ten minutes to the other side of the lake, a place I like to drive to where I can walk along the water's edge or sit and read. At night, looking across, you see a dark landscape dotted with lights from the homes on the gentle, rolling hillside.

Tuesday 12 March

More tests today to check the blood. Had a lousy night, panicky at the way things are. Went to surgery, had ear syringed – tiny spot of blood. What a drag this sinus problem is. I'm told I should check with an ear, nose and throat doctor when back home. Personally, I don't feel that is the way to go: I've been that route before – to no avail – and reckon there must be another approach but I don't know what. After my visit I closed my eyes and dozed for a couple of hours. It's 17 degrees centigrade and a summer-like day in spring. Made a salad lunch and went to Kreuth, sat by the river and read a while, then played the piano for an hour at the *Kuramt* to pick me up. I don't have a headache but I'm glad to get the wig off as it's beginning to be a bit uncomfortable. Thank goodness my own hair is beginning to show signs of improvement. It will still be light at 6.30pm; the season seems to be changing so quickly. This week, for the first time, I am ready to go home and as this is the sixth week, where the treatment starts to make dramatic changes in the system, I know I can expect a day or two of feeling 'under the weather'.

Wednesday 13 March

When I return to London, I'll have to bring all my medication with me. Tom has gone to great lengths through our GP to arrange for someone to give me the daily injections. However, the UK health service has blocked every attempt with rigid rules and regulations – no surprise there. I had warned Dr Fryda of likely difficulties as Tom progressively became frustrated in his enquiries with the NHS, consequently spurring me on to learn how to inject myself.

A great night out with Irene and her friend Cait: their 'final night', as they need to pack up tomorrow night for going home to Ireland early the following morning. We meet at our favourite local restaurant. I take with me an orange, a syringe and a needle, so I can practise my injecting technique as obviously I'm going to need it when I get back to the UK. Fortunately Cait's a nurse so she's in charge. Here are the instructions (should you ever need to inject an orange). First, create a space, i.e. remove cutlery, napkins and any other Bavarian table bric-a-brac likely to hinder the process. Take a glass of water (no point in wasting wine) then assemble needle and syringe. Dip the needle into the water and draw a small amount up into the syringe. Hold the orange firmly in the other hand. Place the needle against orange skin and gently press to insert – at which point, hopefully, you will be sensitive enough to feel the delicate amount of resistance as you pierce the skin. Push the needle in to the required depth; hold it there   then with the thumb steadily depress the syringe to deposit the water into the orange. Gently withdraw the needle. As the evening progresses you will find yourself able to do this whilst eating and drinking your way through a three-course meal. This was definitely our best night out, with more red wine than usual, and a bit of a hoot, as the locals are not accustomed to seeing injections being shot into oranges over dinner (can't think why)!

Thursday 14 March

Another heavenly summer-like day. Tai Chi by the river. Rest of day with Cait and Irene in Rottach-Egern and Tegernsee. Last night was exceptionally good and their packing is ahead of schedule, con-sequently we fit in another dinner at the *Gasthof* over the bridge. Grand night!

Friday 15 March

Group photo with Dr Fryda, her assistant Frau Tippolt, Irene, Cait and me. Off they go, back to Ireland looking radiant and very happy. Clean the kitchen and look forward to a long walk.

Saturday 16 March

Another sunny day. Shampooed hair and for the first time there is no bald patch after drying. Alleluia! Bought Dr Fryda a 75th-birthday present for next Friday. Took a long walk and back for a late lunch feeling good. I am a little apprehensive about the final week seven.

Tuesday 19 March

Second attempt and success at self-injection with the 'team' looking on. Lots of irritation from Dr Fryda at my left-handed handling of the syringe. 'It looks *so* awkward!' she shrieked. Frau Tippolt supervised – just about managing to restrain herself from showing me how to do it. We've had *regen* (rain) all day (thank God I know a *few* more words after all this time). I got something from the *Apotheke* for my stuffed up sinuses. Tomorrow is the day for blood test results. Dr Fryda says it will be good if the markers have gone down, but it's possible they'll still be up and not to worry as that can also be normal at this early stage. I am watching the men's world skating championships and the rain beats down non-stop on the skylight.

Wednesday 20 March

Flights home have proved difficult with the Easter holiday, so I must return after Easter, on 3 April. Not perfect, but should my results arrive late, I'd rather be here for them, than back in the UK. Into the surgery this morning and no results yet. Dr Fryda watched me do my own injection, getting *very* frustrated at my style and instructing me all the time. As my technique becomes more and more accomplished, despite it being shall we say 'left-handed and rather unique', I've grown enormously in confidence and refuse to be put off, smiling smugly as I withdraw the needle with a '… there we are!' She rolls her eyes upwards. There are always such good feelings from her and she so wants me to be well. I feel high on the idea of just one week of treatment left and I'm on the phone to the hairdresser back home in the hope of salvation. Joni Mitchell's recent album is playing and the rain is pissing down outside whilst I have a big sort-out, leaving less for next week when I can concentrate on packing up.

Friday 22 March

My marker is down. Yesssss! Fantastic news. Dr Fryda is thrilled. She is also thrilled with the necklace I have given her for her birthday and I am nothing short of delirious and reeling with delight at the results. It's *so* good. This afternoon, after a large lunch I went over the pass into Austria to the Swarovsky crystal factory and bought Jane, my god-daughter, a birthday present and some gifts for home – still celebrating my results! The rain has continued unabated since Monday evening, but the return journey over Achensee and the mountains at 5pm was amazing. The clouds dropped down over the road, the temperature dropped from five degrees to minus two and as I crossed the Austrian border back into Germany, I saw the snow had obviously followed me on the outward journey a few hours earlier. Now, after a further drop to minus five, the snow was rapidly settling on the roads. The whole experience was ghostly, an amazing contrast to earlier and typical of the sudden changes in the mountains. Back in my apartment now and outside the snow getting deeper by the minute.

Saturday 23 March

Snow, snow, snow. I write at midday and there is a blizzard of horizontal snow. Best to stay holed up. Fortunately I have over-catered for these remaining days. Not long to go. I feel ready now and I'm so looking forward to getting back to Tom, Robert and Alex, family, friends and home.

Tuesday 2 April

My last visit at the surgery has been one of hugs, flowers and happy farewells. Already packed, and this evening Herr and Frau Franck, with their daughter and son-in-law, entertained me to dinner. I've grown very fond of the family, gradually managing to speak better

German, helped by Frau Franck's daughter who translates my English very well. They've all been so kind and the little touches – like the weekly gift of freshly laid eggs – will be greatly missed.

The following morning Herr Franck helped me load the car. Although Tom had already taken home some of my clothes the suitcases were heavy with supplies that I couldn't obtain at home – especially the good German coffee and fine wholegrain baking flour. I drove to Munich airport and on arrival checked in and was about to buy a newspaper when a copy of *Hello* magazine caught my eye. On the cover was a picture of Koo Stark, the actress and photographer who had recently had a mastectomy. The article told of how she had experienced delay in diagnosis in the UK and was being treated in the USA where she had her operation. Like me, her prime concern was for her health and not a reconstruction. Her surgeon said it was usual to remove 9 lymph nodes, but Koo had 15 removed. I had 21 taken and this set me wondering why the number of lymph nodes removed should vary so much. There appeared to be no consensus of opinion. Because cancer was found in Koo's lymph nodes, she was to have chemotherapy. Encouragingly, in the article she went on to say, 'I don't think losing a breast is anything to be ashamed of. I don't feel less feminine and I don't think any woman who loses a bosom should feel she is unattractive.' Wonderful, inspiring stuff – but, several months down the line, the reality of living with a mastectomy didn't leave me, or, I suspected, many other women, feeling like this. I knew I must look much further into breast cancer, write about both my experience and my concern that the medical establishment and cancer research appear to be a 'closed shop', not giving much attention to cause, prevention, or how to unravel cancer and reverse its process in order to prevent this barbaric, drastic surgery being performed on women.

Here the diary ended, to be briefly resumed in August, a few months later. Meanwhile, back at home in the UK, the daily regime of injections and supplements helped me both physically and mentally to feel I was playing a continuing role in bringing myself back to health. My GP was highly cooperative in my request for blood tests and sympathetic to the fact that continuing with a treatment not recognized in this country meant that I was virtually on my own. This sense of being on my own was hard sometimes, but generally I put my mind to creating and adapting recipes to make the diet more interesting and trying to regain as normal a life as possible: I found acupuncture, healing and meditation essential. After an initial disaster at the hairdressers, when my hair turned vibrant red, I enrolled the help of Gerard, my stylist, and traced my former colourist, Mikko, who put his magic skills to work to revive the normal colour in my rapidly growing, now unusually curly hair. The quality of the new hair was delicate and it was another three years before it fully returned to its former condition. The PR meetings for the launch of Tom's book in the autumn were a helpful distraction, as were my students and occasional visits to the theatre in London's West End, to see them at work. Soon it was August and I was ready to return to Germany for a six-month check. By now the menopause had completely arrived and I was far from feeling 'serene'.

7 Changes – The Quest Begins

Back to Germany for ten days for a six-month check-up. There's hardly any accommodation available, so I take a room in a house. Self-contained domesticity, again.

Sunday 4 August

From the window I can see nothing except green trees dripping with rain with the weather more like April and cold – 11 degrees. This newly kitted out room is like a doll's house. 'Compact' would be an understatement. I almost expected to hear a fanfare as the owner, Frau Neumann, dramatically flung open the double doors of what looked like a wardrobe to reveal … a kitchen. Her sweeping gesture conjured up the launching of a ship: I could almost hear the sound of a champagne bottle crashing on the hob, and had to stop myself from saying, 'I name this the wardrobe kitchen – God bless all who cook in her!'

Contemplating life and what I need to do next feels rather like stepping off the pavement just as a lorry comes by. Anyhow, what *is it* that I want – to become a sex goddess at 50-something with one breast? Get a tattoo? I'm totally perplexed with myself.

Tuesday 6 August

At Dr Fryda's surgery today I managed to make her understand how, eleven months after the operation, I've not come to terms with looking at myself naked with a missing breast. 'Tom has no problem with you being without a breast; what are you worried about?' she asked. 'That isn't the point,' I said. 'It's missing and I feel empty, it's a part of me as a woman, and I feel dreadful about it. On a good day I can push the thoughts aside, but every night and every morning this empty space stares back at me, and I hate it.' She thought for a moment, then said, 'It is a big effort at my age to keep looking good, as for you, I do not *know*, but I can imagine how I would feel – and it must be terrible.' Her attitude is always sensitive yet direct, whilst her knowledge is remarkable. The feeling that the healing process is one of partnership is undoubtedly one of the prime motivators of my self-empowerment and the importance of this can never be overestimated. I know I must be patient just now.

Thursday 8 August

As I write, there's a continual roar from the traffic on its way to Austria. I feel in transit here in more ways than one. Unfortunately this trip has broken up my new London routine of going to the gym and I'm not pleased with the restricted accommodation either. The best I can do is put on a raincoat, take an umbrella and walk for an hour whilst learning some more German on the Walkman. I wait for Tom's call with the faxed results of the tests I had taken in London last week. Must have supper in a quiet restaurant to read at least fifty pages of Tom's manuscript *The Boiled Frog Syndrome* – subtitled *Your Health and the Built Environment* – and feel, rather eerily, that if I had known beforehand about everything in his book, I might have prevented myself from getting breast cancer. Who knows? Just another of life's funny twists.

Eating out is difficult, everywhere is busy and it's often tricky to avoid added sugar or refined ingredients. I remember in the past thinking how picky some people can be in restaurants – well now

I'm one of them. Sometimes the challenge to be inventive with my diet is almost inspiring and at other times I feel I'm eating to an absolute regime. I have greatly reduced the amount of time spent juicing which is a great relief as I'm no longer wading through mountains of carrots. Going away for even a day means being armed with pills, snacks, water, tea bags, etc. and the very act of travelling minimally is a thing of the past. In fact, on this trip the suitcase was mainly taken up with a mini kitchen. The worst nightmare is whether to put all this culinary equipment in hand-luggage or the hold, knowing that every item is essential. And what if some gets lost? These newly found neurotic tendencies leave me feeling incredulous about myself. The days of packing a few choice items of clothing in hand-luggage seem well and truly over and I suspect part of the problem is that I believe the 'real me' is still 20-something and a free spirit that requires little more than the wind in her hair. Here we reach a deeply sore point as my formerly long, thick hair is still recovering. How callously we women are treated. Throughout history, the shaving of women's heads has been used as a punishment and humiliation, whether it was inflicted on the women branded as witches in the Middle Ages, or the French women who – as mentioned earlier – were condemned as traitors after the Second World War. The story of Samson and the consequences of his hair loss are completely understandable to me. I wonder how it must feel for a man to lose a testicle and all his hair at the same time; much the same I guess – disastrous.

Friday 16 August

I am home in London, back two weeks, and writing this now because things in Germany improved to such an extent that I didn't need to write. Much of the anger I had been feeling during my stay there was later quelled by the unexpected, joyous company of women. By an extraordinary coincidence whilst idly looking in a dress shop nearby, I complimented the assistant on her good English, to which she replied that she practised with a friend of hers who was an opera singer. My ears pricked up at this as I have worked with many opera singers, so I asked who that might be. When she told me, I laughed as I knew her friend well and so we struck up a friendship and had much to talk about. After a few days I moved away from the 'kitchen in a wardrobe' to a much quieter and more spacious place. I stayed in the home of Frau Dimond who used part of her large house for holiday apartments. She was an elderly woman of indefinable age, with a magical quality about her; like a breath of fresh air, she spoke fluent English and I loved our chatter. Her long grey hair was pulled straight back in a chignon and, whether doing housework or relaxing, she made the best of her appearance. There was the quality of a young girl about the way she wore her dresses and jewellery, her tiny feet trimmed with scarlet nail varnish as if she were indulging her 'Aphrodite' qualities to a level of pleasure that I had lost. This was totally in keeping with the magic scenery, soft grass, sweeping rivers and velvet green mountains – all so different from living the London life where injections, grinding machines, juicers and the like were top priority. After the housework, Frau Dimond often reclined on the broad balcony to read whilst surrounded by the peaceful sounds of nature. Rooted in nature! That's what I miss in the chaos of London. How can I aspire to the delightful freedom of Frau Dimond whilst having to travel on public transport in London: an assault course immersed in pollution?

Back to the state of the body. Generally, Dr Fryda is pleased with my progress, but disappointed that the adrenaline is still way down and that it could take another six or seven months to recover. The exercise in the gym leaves me with a headache, I feel lacking in energy and must quit for a while. I have absolutely no desire to do anything active or meaningful. What is it about the menopause? I am watching changes in my body and I wonder why it seems to be a stage in a woman's life that no one really wants to talk about. Is there in existence a book that gives the complete A–Z of the menopause and all its symptoms? I have dipped into endless information about diet and supplements, but I'm doing all those things anyway, and yet nothing helps. The side effects of tamoxifen appear to be glossed over by the doctors, with emphasis only on the benefits. A gynaecologist in London just happened to say that the effects of tamoxifen will continue in the body for six months after stopping taking it, which I find very disturbing.

Beyond the diary of August 2002, and throughout the following year, I had to deal with the menopause, a lack of energy, sinus problems with an almost continual lack of taste and smell and, at times, almost hourly hot flushes. The homeopath I visited wasn't able to help. In a supreme effort to 'blow away' my lethargy, I started tennis training, only to develop tennis elbow, and had to stop. Almost every turning presented a setback until I decided to find supplements to help deal with the problems, and at the same time I began reflexology sessions with Tony Porter, a well-known international reflexologist. This was a tremendous boost and by April 2003, my visit to Germany showed that, at last, my adrenaline was registering a healthy amount. During my stay, however, I had to take antibiotics and spent a couple of days in bed, thoroughly knocked out with another attack of sinusitis. On my return to London, I took the advice of a friend of ours, Tad Mann – an American author and astrologer – to contact Joan Lykke in Denmark, a complex homeopath who uses Vega testing for diagnosis. After all these years, complex homeopathy seemed an unlikely solution to such a chronic problem, but by now I was desperate, and vowed to rid myself of any lurking illness that might hinder my regaining full health.

The most subtle medicine

Nothing short of miraculous. Within two weeks of taking Joan Lykke's treatment, all the symptoms had disappeared and by early June both my taste and smell returned to such an extent that I realized they'd been cut off for years. At times, my new-found senses were almost overwhelming – it was an utter delight and has remained so ever since. This was the beginning of a steady clearing process throughout the system and gradually the headaches became lighter.

Perhaps the most important revelation was that after all I had gone through up to now, the gravity that generally surrounds cancer, and the fact that Dr Fryda's regenerating treatment had allowed my system to right itself, finally brought me to a place where I was clearing a 14-year-old persistent physical aggravation, with a few innocent drops of complex homeopathy. It was another extraordinary proof of the body making what seemed to be a very small adjustment in order to create an overwhelming return to health. It echoed all that I find in my work with my students' voices – that the line between a 'good' sound and a 'poor' sound is, so often, very small. As the upward trend continued, I came across Leslie Kenton's book *Passage to Power*. This book is still the best I know for explaining and dealing easily with many health problems women may encounter, particularly at the menopause. At last I found the benefit of natural remedies, and confirmation of my belief that HRT wasn't the answer for me. I'd yet to find a solution to the hot flushes which came and went – often in reaction to a minute change in the weather – my body behaving like some super-sensitive barometer.

Talking to other women was an enormous help and I discovered that a major concern for women who've had breast cancer is the possible connection of menopausal symptoms to the illness. Clearly the menopause is a time of confusion when, after the breast cancer treatment is over, women are often very alone to cope with menopausal problems, many having difficulty in finding experienced and wise counsellors.

Ready to begin anew

Looking back on my initial treatment in London, I was spurred on to expose the half-truths of the diagnosis and treatment of breast cancer. At present we undergo the 'standard treatment' only to be left to get on with life afterwards, as if nothing has happened to us. Then, when we reach the menopause, we are expected to cope with it like 'normal' women, when everything that has been done to our bodies in treating the cancer has changed our 'normality'. It appalled me to think that my bright, beautiful, young women friends and students should ever suffer the same crude treatment that I and millions of other women have had to experience: we all deserve far better than this. Now was the time to make some major changes in my life.

And so I began with a new-found strength on the next round of research, but this time working in a state of recovery rather than illness. With my women friends at the front of my mind, and with their encouragement, I drove on in my quest to give something back and share the discoveries that might help others. Above all, I wanted to find information on how to help prevent this disease.

PART TWO

The Politics Of Cancer

I will prevent disease whenever I can, for prevention is preferable to cure.

Hippocratic Oath
(Modern Version by Dr Louis Lasagna, 1964)

A third of European cancer patients are using complementary and alternative therapies... Given their popularity, governments should rethink the way these treatments are regulated.

Annals of Oncology 2005
(According to members of the European Oncology Nursing
Society, 3 February 2005)

8 Mammography and Radiation

I began my research by looking into mammograms, as I was highly suspicious of their role in my breast cancer – after all, my last mammogram in 2001 had been followed by the swift appearance of a lump, which two doctors had diagnosed as a cyst when it was actually cancer. Instinctively, I felt that it was not a coincidence that the cancer had appeared so soon after having a mammogram. Had the mammogram been instrumental in its appearance?

NHS breast screening

The NHS Breast Screening Programme was set up in 1988 by the Department of Health. According to information published by Breast Cancer Relief in January 2004, the NHS was screening 1,500,000 women every year, with over 90 breast screening units each inviting an average of 45,000 women for screening each year. The screening was every 3 years for women aged 50–64, and it was planned to extend this to age 70 by 2004. Beyond the age of 65, women were encouraged to make their own appointments.[1]

A search of the NHS Breast Screening Programme website in May 2006 found much the same information and confirmed that the age range for screening had now extended to age 70. It explained that women under 50 are not offered routine screening because mammograms are not as effective in premenopausal women.[2]

Breast screening: the questions

'Understanding Breast Screening' was a booklet sent to me from the NHS Breast Screening Programme in 2004. In the section 'Common Questions About Breast Cancer Screening' it asks 'Why are women under 50 not screened?' and then explains that breast cancer is rare in women under 50 and tells us that 50 is the average age for the menopause in the UK. At the menopause, mammograms can see what goes on in the breast tissue more easily than in younger women whose breast tissue is different and not suitable for the mammogram procedure. 'Breast cancer is rare in women under 50' does not seem to me to be a realistic assessment of the situation in either 2004 or 2006. Furthermore, the fact that younger women cannot be screened because their breast tissue doesn't suit the machinery seems lacking to say the least.

Clearly it was time to look more deeply into the subject so I went to the British Library and began my research. There I discovered that the unfamiliar world of science that I was entering has a pecking order and that only the so-called 'serious' research is really looked upon as being of any use. It did not take long for me to find that amongst this serious research there was much more evidence about the uncertainty of mammograms than I could ever have imagined. Scientific papers emerged with titles such as 'Another round in the mammography controversy'; 'Mammography at a crossroad. How do physicians reconcile conflicting study results with the biologic truths of breast cancer?'; 'Amid controversy, task force recommends more widespread use of mammograms'; 'Making up your own minds about mammograms'; 'False positive screening with mammograms', and 'Risk of subsequent breast cancer in relation to characteristics of screening mammograms from women less than 50 years of age'.

These were just a few of the reports which made me realize that I had to start writing – and fast.

I noted with interest that in the national publicity for mammograms on television and in the newspapers in the UK, the woman being prepared for the mammogram is always pictured from behind while the radiographer stands beside her, facing the camera. This image suggests that a standard procedure is about to take place, not unlike having an ordinary X-ray taken. However, unlike the ordinary X-ray, there is a big difference when undergoing a mammogram. The scene we are shown masks what is really going on, and if we were to see the full frontal and side views of the process, it would not be a pretty sight.

Breast screening: the mammogram

'Breast screening' means having a mammogram. Unless you have already had a mammogram, you – and particularly the men in your family – will probably have little or no idea of what is involved. Talking to friends beneath the 50-year-old threshold and therefore not old enough to be automatically offered a mammogram, I found them astonishingly ignorant; but then in hindsight, so was I.

In essence, breast screening seems to work on the principle of no pain, no gain. My experience and that of many others seems to be that the more the breast is squashed the better the chances of producing a clearer image. Prior to my breast cancer, the few routine mammograms that I had were not pleasant and I doubt that any woman, unless she has sadomasochistic tendencies, could say it is a pleasant experience. The leaflet published in the UK in 2003 by the Department of Health tells us that some women find it uncomfortable, others experience pain whilst the procedure lasts, and for a small number of women the pain continues for some time after. The latest information attempts to be a little more realistic and tells us that *most* women find it uncomfortable and a few quite painful. The point is also made that, like other medical tests, mammography is not 100 per cent accurate and that it is calculated that approximately 7 per cent of breast cancers are not visible on X-rays, therefore women should be encouraged to be continually breast aware.[3] This information must leave many women feeling uncertain about the accuracy of the test and rather apprehensive about the likely pain or discomfort. The medical establishment constantly reminds us of the importance of mammograms for diagnosing breast cancer, but if we were given all the information about the limitations and the possible after-effects, many women might seriously think twice before having a mammogram.

The mammogram procedure

First you undress to the waist. The mammogram machine has four transparent plastic plates sometimes referred to as 'paddles'. Standing in front of the machine you're then asked to place one breast on the plate lying directly in front of you. It is rather strange to be able to view your own breast as a 'body part' which is how it now looks. The top plate is then brought down onto the breast, pressing the breast into a flat shape which bears an uncanny resemblance to the shrink-wrapped chicken breasts we find in a supermarket meat freezer. It hardly needs saying that this is the point where, so we are told in the most recent official information, most women find it uncomfortable and a few quite painful. Then the radiographer goes away behind a protective screen to view the picture of the breast. If the picture is not showing clearly all that she would like to see, the radiographer will return and place the breast more appropriately on the plate, sometimes asking you to push up as close to the plate as possible with every part of the breast pressed forward on to it, at which point it may be necessary to squeeze the plates even closer together. The radiographer may reassure you that it will only be uncomfortable for a short time – and being women we tend to tolerate the pain or discomfort by telling ourselves that it's all to the good. The radiographer then goes back behind the protective screen and asks you to hold your breath and keep as still as possible. A quick shot of radiation and the image has been taken.

However, this is not the end: the whole procedure is repeated with the same breast now being squashed from side to side with further plates which resemble an upright 'transparent' sandwich-toaster. The procedures are then repeated on the other breast.

My own experience of mammograms

Following previous mammograms I had experienced some tenderness in my breasts, but the results had been clear. Just before the very last mammogram in April 2001, neither the doctor nor I could feel any lumps in either breast, nor was there any tenderness, but after the mammogram my left breast became constantly tender and, just a short time afterwards, the lump appeared. We are told that cancerous lumps are very rarely painful; however this one, rather like a cyst, *was* painful and at the same time I correctly sensed it was something different.

Remarkably, the results of this mammogram had shown no problems and I was given the all-clear, so the tenderness and rapid appearance of the lump led me to conclude that the mammogram had played a role in its manifestation. Interestingly, no NHS doctor involved in my further treatment has ever either refuted or condoned my belief that this was the case. Instead, it has been met with silence. On a check-up visit to the hospital a year after my breast cancer operation, I was told I must have a mammogram. Having an annual mammogram after having breast cancer is quite usual. I refused, making it very clear that I'd never have one again. I accepted the ultrasound examination as an alternative, convinced by then that all examinations using radiation and electromagnetic fields are hazardous to a greater or lesser degree.

I had to question why this brutal mammogram procedure is believed to be suitable for such a delicate thing as the breast? I knew that in my professional voice work, if I adopted such a harsh, physical approach, it would be completely destructive. My suspicions about the dangers were soon to be confirmed.

Mammograms: the facts

It seems that where mammograms are concerned there are greater risks involved than we are led to believe. The cost to our health in having a mammogram test varies from woman to woman with nobody knowing for certain how each individual will react. It becomes a gamble in which otherwise healthy women may be putting themselves at risk.

In the USA, Bill Sturgeon of Petrolia, a Food and Drug Administration (FDA) certified medical device manufacturer, and health and science writer for the Humboldt Senior Resource Centre, reported:

> In addition to the cumulative damage incurred from the mammographic penetrating radiation, cancer cells, if present in the breast as a tumour, can possibly be spread from being squashed in the mammogram machine. As for 'early detection' the malignant tumour disclosed by a mammogram is, on average, seven or eight years old already! [4]

Michael Baum, Emeritus Professor of Surgery and visiting Professor of Humanities at University College London, chairs one of the largest breast cancer trials worldwide and set up the NHS Breast Screening Programme in the south-east of England in 1987. After leaving the programme he became an outspoken critic of mammography. His concerns over screening and breast cancer are clear, whether it is a matter of false alarms and over-treatment or what he describes as a false promise from the NHS screening programme which suggests that if you catch breast cancer early, your breast can be saved. He says that this is not the truth and women are pressurized into screening, but they are not being fully informed about the risks. He said, 'The agents of the state say I am a maverick but I am at the sharp end and I can see the casualties of screening.'[5]

Professor Baum is not alone in his misgivings about the screening for breast cancer. The following statistics do not give any reassurances that mammograms are in our best interests, especially given the fact that they are deemed unsuitable for young women. This being the case, and knowing that the NHS offers mammograms for women age 50 to 70, how much *are* they helping to detect breast cancer?

> [Mammography] will reduce the risk of death from breast cancer by approximately 30 per cent in women over 50 years old ... [Mammography] is limited in that cancer, like breast tissue, appears white on the X-ray. [6]

In her book *Passage to Power*, Lesley Kenton brings our attention to a report entitled 'Breast Scans Boost Risk of Cancer Death' which in 1991 became the headline of an article in *The Times* informing us that 'Middle-aged women who have regular mammograms are more likely to die from breast cancer than women who are not screened, according to dramatic new research.' [7]

In 2006, we saw no change in our welfare following this devastating evidence. Breast scans are more prevalent now than ever before. Why? With all this evidence why does a new hospital wing dealing with breast cancer install mammography equipment? As far as I am aware, there is not one hospital dealing with breast cancer that doesn't regularly use mammography as the first call in diagnosis.

Equally worrying is the research at the University of Gottingen by Dr Malis Frankenberg-Schwager, who is concerned that the low energy X-rays used in mammograms are putting women who are genetically predisposed to breast cancer at risk. This reinforces the findings of other research into the dangers of extremely low electromagnetic fields which mimic the low electrical pulses within the human body. (We are generally led to believe that only high voltage is dangerous.) It appears that mammograms are nearly three times more likely to cause genes to mutate compared to conventional

X-rays and, according to Dr Frankenberg-Schwager, a typical 4 milligray mammogram could damage the genes in 16 out of every 100 million cells: one in 200 women have mutations of the BRCA1 and BRCA2 gene linked to breast cancer. Worse still, those who *know* they are at risk are encouraged to have annual mammogram check-ups despite the *New Scientist* magazine reporting that for these women 'mammograms could therefore further increase their risk of the disease.'[8]

However, the response on BBC Ceefax in 2002 by Dr Roger Cox of the UK's National Radiological Protection Board (NRPB) was: 'I don't believe these findings have any implications for breast cancer screening in general.' As for women genetically at risk, he didn't suggest ruling out mammograms, but thought they probably should be viewed as individual cases.[9] Meanwhile, increasingly we hear of women who are genetically at risk having surgery for double mastectomies as a precaution against breast cancer.

Yet another report two years later on the BBC in 2004 told us that a study in Belfast by Richard Kennedy drew attention to the risk of regular mammograms for those at high risk with gene mutations. Kennedy is reported as saying, 'These women have a choice between surgery and regular screening and they must be aware of the risks of both.'[10]

Are you one of these high-risk women? If you are, then you are clearly being told that the choice is yours and either way involves risks. The results of studies such as that carried out in Belfast and Dr Frankenberg-Schwager's earlier research, leave women at a loss as to what to do for the best, highlighting the current unsatisfactory state of screening.

The National Radiological Protection Board (NRPB)[11]

In recent years it has become increasingly evident that the governments of many so-called 'civilized' countries are prepared neither to be honest nor to allow their citizens to make their own, well-informed decisions. It is vital that we do, especially where breast cancer is concerned – not only for the sake of women and men now, but for future generations. The National Radiological Protection Board (NRPB), a UK Government body, funded by the UK taxpayer, is supposedly there to protect us from the adverse effects of radiation. Yet it has continually taken the stance of ignoring the rigorous scientific research from other countries which indicates the harmful effects of radiation, whether it be from mobile phones, mobile phone aerial-masts, TETRA masts or overhead power lines and other potential radiation hazards, saying that they don't believe that there is any evidence of these being harmful – the same response as they gave to Dr Frankenberg-Schwager's research. Meanwhile, the general public continues to finance the NRPB which arrogantly dismisses the highest calibre of worldwide scientific research. Simon Best edits and publishes *Electromagnetic Hazard and Therapy* and in the *Institute for Complementary Medicine Journal* he reviewed the NRPB report published in January 2003 in an article entitled 'Health Effects from Radiofrequency Electromagnetic Fields'. He said, 'The NRPB still seem to consider people as dead slabs of meat with a built in cooling system (the circulating blood). They have yet to acknowledge the idea of "life energies" based on science, giving the impression that they are merely pandering to industry demands and government agendas.'

Throughout my research, a picture has emerged revealing that in breast cancer there appears to be a delicate but crucial 'tipping-point' that varies from woman to woman, at which depletions in the body – however insignificant they may look in the general picture – create a window where we might become vulnerable to breast cancer. Rather like the medical establishment who support cut, poison and burn, the NRPB ignores this delicate issue of variation in a woman's body. The NRPB says that a mammogram exposes you to the same amount of radiation as you would receive as natural background radiation over a few months. This seems an incredibly vague method of quantifying the dosage. The very idea of having a few months of radiation piled up and then administered in one shot of a mammogram is all right then? In addition there is no consideration given to the varying quality and maintenance of the equipment being used.

The issue of out-of-date equipment was raised in January 2004 in a study titled 'Best before – An Investigation into the Crumbling State of NHS Hospitals and Equipment'. The gist of the report was that, according to research, 'Out of date and "patched up" NHS equipment is putting patients' lives at risk. The backlog of repairs has reached £3.4 billion with the diagnosis and treatment of diseases delayed as a result.'[12] Liberal Democrat Member of Parliament Paul Burstow, who put together the dossier taken from the study, warned: 'Equipment that is past its "best before" date undermines quality care.' This presumably includes mammography. The UK has a large variety of different screening machines and each machine can give slightly different readings. Consequently, it is not conducive to safe and accurate readings to have operators moving from one machine to another. How would we know how competent and sensitive the radiographer is or how well the machinery is maintained?

The following extract from a paper published in *Radiographics 2003*, the journal of the Radiological Society of North America, gives us a very clear indication that the quality of the results of a mammogram is dependent on the best and most highly maintained machines. To have a mammogram taken as accurately as possible, you require a radiographer capable of performing with meticulous attention to every detail when they position the breast.

> Mammography is the standard of reference for the detection of breast carcinoma, yet 10%–30% of breast carcinomas may be missed at mammography. Possible causes for the missed breast cancers include dense parenchyma obscuring a lesion, poor positioning or technique, perception error, incorrect interpretation of a suspect finding, subtle features of malignancy, and slow

growth of a lesion. Recent studies have emphasized the use of alternative imaging modalities to detect and diagnose breast carcinoma, including ultrasonography (US), magnetic resonance imaging, and nuclear medicine studies. However the radiologist can take a number of steps that will significantly enhance the accuracy of image interpretation at mammography and decrease the false-negative rate.[13]

Research on the link between radiation and cancer

According to research published in *The Lancet* in 2004, there is no safe minimum threshold beneath which radiation might induce cancer. Diagnostic X-rays may induce some cancers to the equivalent of 700 cases a year in the UK. CT scans, barium enemas and hip and pelvis X-rays are said to contribute highly. According to the authors these figures would naturally reduce if the radiation dose were less, or there were less frequent exposures to X-rays.[14]

With this kind of information at hand, it is not surprising to learn that US scientists have recently found that pregnant women having dental X-rays are three times more likely to give birth to an underweight full-term baby. Other research from the US recently informed us that:

> Full body scans expose people to similar levels of radiation as atomic bombs used on Hiroshima. Scientists say CT or computed tomography scans use ionizing radiation to take pictures of the inside of the body and can detect things like cancer. But they can also cause cancer, US scientists at Columbia University say in the journal *Radiology*. They warned healthy people not to seek full-body CT scans as part of their health check-ups. [15]

The mammogram that I underwent just before the cancerous lump appeared was quite straightforward although rather painful. The radiographer appeared to be efficient and didn't waste any time with the procedure, mentioning that she hoped to be going on holiday the next day.

Later, it was pointed out to me by my surgeon at the Royal Marsden Hospital that this mammogram, which I believe was the turning point in the cancerous lump arriving, was taken on a much older machine than the one at the Royal Marsden. We viewed the pictures from both mammogram machines to find that there was a significant variation in the general quality, the older one being less distinct.

The importance of scientific evidence

Between 1980 and 1988 The Canadian National Breast Cancer Screening Study tracked 50,000 women in their forties: half received periodic mammograms; the other half received periodic physical examinations only. The results showed that:

> ... the increased risk of death from breast cancer for women undergoing mammography was reported to be a full 36% ... over those who received only the physical examination. The director of the study observed: 'One potential problem was that surgery, the anaesthetic and radiotherapy involved in treating women with breast cancer were interfering with immunity. [As a result] the initial radiation and surgery to remove tiny breast lumps discovered by mammograms may make secondary cancers elsewhere grow faster ... You may find the cancers earlier (with mammography), but the women are still going to die. Modern treatment does not work for these early cancers.[16]

This gloomy outlook is confirmed by top scientists in cancer research who continue to suggest that mammograms are unsafe, putting women's health and lives at risk. As I discovered, safer and much more efficient ways of breast screening are available, but very few women are told of these methods by the medical profession because the standard practice is to use the mammogram. Why? These are very urgent questions to be answered by the medical profession. How many more alarm calls do they need before they wake up to the reality of the situation? When will the Establishment take as much care of their patients as they do of their reputations and the niceties of professional etiquette? The price of failing to act upon the hard, scientific evidence revealing the risks associated with mammograms is paid with human lives. Why are so many reports that clearly show positive findings then watered down by caveats? Is this because the experts do not have the courage to publish the true results, or do they prefer to sit on the fence to avoid upsetting their more orthodox peers or their conservative bosses? Who makes the final decision as to how the vital research is implemented or ignored? In chapter 14 'Alternatives to Mammography' we will see what happens when reports show very clear, positive findings and then summarize by sitting on the fence (*see* page 180). All of this is deeply disturbing when there are safer methods to be found.

9 Tamoxifen and Similar Drugs

The dilemma

In the same way that mammographic screening for breast cancer carries potential health risks, so too do the drugs used in the treatment of breast cancer. We do not have much choice in this – the drugs we are offered are highly toxic, even potentially carcinogenic and carry risks for the rest of our health. This is not a choice.

A National Cancer Institute fact sheet tells us that tamoxifen has been in use for more than twenty years. It appears that tamoxifen was developed in the UK and first used to fight breast cancer at the Christie Hospital in Manchester, England in 1969. We are informed that the drug is cheap and helps prevent the cancer coming back after the initial surgery. By working against the effects of the body's oestrogen, tamoxifen is intended to slow down or stop the growth of cancer cells and this would be a valid reason to consider taking it.

Many women like myself are led by standard medical practice to believe that the overriding issue in the most common type of oestrogen receptor positive breast cancer is to get the oestrogen as low as possible, and the principal, most widely used drug for this in many parts of the world is tamoxifen. I know that I panicked when

I decided to take it, as I had been bombarded with information about the dangers of high oestrogen in late-menopausal women. Consequently, after abandoning chemotherapy, I continued taking tamoxifen in the hope that it was doing some good. Once I began my restorative treatment in Germany and learned that cancer is a systemic disease, I was given the choice of continuing with tamoxifen, or stopping. I gradually withdrew after a total of nine to ten months.

Risks

The information available on tamoxifen is somewhat surprising and enough to cause total confusion to any of us reading it, regardless of whether we have breast cancer or not. The website of the National Cancer Institute (NCI), informs us that:

> ... there are risks associated with tamoxifen. Some are even life-threatening. The decision to take tamoxifen is an individual one: some women experience irregular menstrual periods, headaches, fatigue, nausea and/or vomiting, vaginal dryness or itching, irritation of the skin around the vagina and skin rash ... tamoxifen increases the risk of two types of cancer that can develop in the uterus: endometrial cancer, which arises in the lining of the uterus, and uterine sarcoma, which arises in the wall of the uterus. Most of the endometrial cancers that have occurred in women taking tamoxifen have been found in the early stages, and the treatment has usually been effective ... There is a small increase in the number of blood clots ... an increased chance of stroke ... increased risk of cataracts ... possible increase in cancers of the digestive tract.
>
> The ideal length of treatment is not known.[1]

Risks in men

Tamoxifen is also used to treat men with breast cancer. The NCI fact sheet points out that men taking tamoxifen 'may experience headaches, nausea and/or vomiting, skin rash, impotence, or a decrease in sexual interest.' Whilst pointing out that it can cause impotence in men, unfortunately it doesn't appear to point out the same for women, despite some women complaining that tamoxifen causes loss of libido.

Dosage

There seems to be confusion amongst the medical profession as to the length of time a patient should receive tamoxifen. Still, after all these years the length of time considered most appropriate varies. The original plan appears to have been to give tamoxifen for five years, but in recent years the medical profession has become uncertain about this. There was quite a lot of publicity a few years ago which clearly suggested that it would be better to lower the period from five years to about eighteen months or two years. But there does not appear to be a clear rule. I have heard of many women who are still being told by their doctors to take it for five years whilst others are told different, varying amounts of time. It is quite clear that despite its having been in use for more than 30 years, the ideal length of treatment is still unknown.

How this affects those of us who take it is, likewise, not known. Rather like the mammogram controversy, it would be logical to assume that the effects of long-term usage will vary from woman to woman. As tamoxifen, like all breast cancer drugs, is toxic, it would surely be common sense to ask what the *safe* length of time is. If taking these drugs for a longer length of time means that we can prevent a recurrence of breast cancer, then we might reasonably assume that long-term usage could mean five years. But as tamoxifen and other breast cancer drugs are so toxic, it follows that this longer length of time would increase the risk to the rest of our health. Whilst the medical establishment appears to recognize the tragedies of over-treatment, might it not be logical to include carcinogenic drug treatments for breast cancer in this?

Whilst the debate goes on about tamoxifen and the appropriate length of treatment, women naturally look to what else is available. The problem here is that the newer drugs haven't been around long enough for us to know just what the possible long-term side effects may be, and so tamoxifen is often used in preference simply because it has been here longer.

Menopause symptoms

Research indicates that menopause symptoms will be much greater in many women if they take tamoxifen. Many women on tamoxifen and similar drugs are then given hormone replacement therapy (HRT) to counter the menopausal problems created by the artificial lowering of the oestrogens. Despite research which, years ago, assured us it was safe to use, more recent research now shows HRT to be dangerous, increasing the risk of developing heart disease and cancer. Other research, however, advocates the use of natural oestrogen and natural progesterone along with tamoxifen.

In many younger women there is the added problem that this artificial method of lowering the body's oestrogens with tamoxifen will produce menopausal symptoms such as hot flashes, irregular periods and a collection of other menopausal-type problems, but according to the NCI fact sheet 'not all women who take tamoxifen will have these symptoms.' As women are generally pursuing careers and putting off having babies until they are older, this treatment must cause concern in younger women, especially those who do not yet have their own children.

Used as a preventative

We are informed by the National Cancer Institute (www.cancer. gov/cancertopics/factsheet/Therapy/tamoxifen) that in 2006 'Tamoxifen continues to be studied for the prevention of breast cancer. It is also being studied in the treatment of several other types of cancer.' This information may lead us to believe that hopefully in the near future, new discoveries for the prevention of breast cancer might yet be made with regard to tamoxifen. Unfortunately many readers may not be aware that such research was already carried out in the 1990s. *The Lancet* points out that two European research teams found no such protective effect from taking tamoxifen, and caution was expressed as to the possible toxic and genotoxic effects of the drug. One of the trials only used women who had previously undergone hysterectomy as the investigators were concerned about the possibility of endometrial cancer arising from taking tamoxifen.[2] One breast care nurse I spoke to said that she saw as many recurrences from breast cancer amongst the women who had taken tamoxifen, as those who had not.

A carcinogen

Apart from the information supplied by the National Cancer Institute (NCI) which points to the increased risks associated with tamoxifen of developing certain cancers (see page 94), the World Health Organization (WHO) has formally designated tamoxifen as a human carcinogen. Dr Samuel Epstein, Emeritus Professor of Environmental and Occupational Medicine, University of Illinois at the Chicago School of Public Health, in 1992 said of tamoxifen: 'The risks to healthy women of a wide range of serious complications, including uterine cancer, fatal liver disease, liver failure, life-threatening blood clots and crippling menopausal symptoms are unacceptable.' In an article entitled 'Breast Cancer Awareness Month and Tamoxifen', Bill Sturgeon reported that Breast Cancer Awareness Month is funded solely by the makers of tamoxifen.[3]

To be informed by the health authorities that there are risks associated with tamoxifen and that 'the decision to take tamoxifen is an individual one', sounds very much as if the medical establishment are offering these drugs knowing full well that the side effects can even be, in their own words, 'life-threatening', thus passing the onus of responsibility onto the woman (or man) whilst at the same time relinquishing their own responsibility for the woman's health.

The toxic effects of tamoxifen and other cancer drugs on our environment must be impossible to calculate. However, in light of the problems already encountered in the environment due to artificial oestrogens from the contraceptive pill passing into the water supply, these breast cancer drugs may pose an even greater threat, especially in view of their carcinogenic properties.

Other similar drugs

Now we can choose from a variety of similar drugs. Some of the newer ones go even further than tamoxifen and try to deplete the body totally of oestrogen. The available information on these other drugs raises important questions. How does the body react when totally deprived of oestrogen? Why would a menopausal or post-menopausal woman want to take such drugs when her body's oestrogens are automatically lowering or have already lowered considerably at this time? During my stay with Dr Fryda, I learned that not all types of oestrogen in the body are bad, the 'good' oestrogen being an essential part of the hormonal system and very necessary to our health.

On one of my hospital visits at the end of 2001, Arimidex was hailed as yet another most exciting breakthrough (*see* page 43). Arimidex (also known as anastrozole) is an oestrogen suppressant drug and has been hailed more than once as the new wonder drug for breast cancer. I wonder how many men and women know that this drug is unsuitable for premenopausal women? The information on Arimidex tells us: 'If you are pregnant or plan to become pregnant, do not take Arimidex. In animal studies, this medication has caused severe birth defects, including incomplete bone formation and low birth weight; it could be poisonous to your unborn child. Arimidex also increases your chances of having a miscarriage or a stillborn baby. If you should accidentally become pregnant, tell your doctor immediately.' Perhaps this is why it is only recommended for post-menopausal women! The list of side effects – including osteoporosis and raised cholesterol – is lengthy and appears very similar to those associated with tamoxifen. Any post-menopausal woman taking this drug is likely to be worried about the possibility of developing osteoporosis.[4] Despite this information, in 2006 Cancer Research is seeking female volunteers to take part in Ibis-2 trials to test this same drug for the *prevention* of breast cancer. Like the trials for prevention with tamoxifen, after some years will there again be dis-ease within the medical establishment, followed by gestures of disapproval from the medical journals as yet again the side effects of such drugs and trials are seen to endanger otherwise healthy women?

Like Arimidex, Herceptin has also been hailed as a wonder drug. Out of the 41,000 women diagnosed with breast cancer in the UK each year, Herceptin is possibly suitable for about 8,200 women and we are warned that about 10 per cent of these shouldn't take the drug because they have an existing heart problem or high blood pressure. The first patient was enrolled for trials of the drug at the end of 2001, so unfortunately other side effects are probably yet to be discovered. Herceptin is already licensed for those who are in the advanced stages of the disease. Those women who receive chemotherapy as well as Herceptin appear to have a much greater risk of heart problems and we are told: 'The incidence and severity of cardiac dysfunction was particularly high in patients who received Herceptin in combination with [the chemotherapy drugs] anthracyclines and cyclophosphamide.' [5] For further information, see the *Ecologist* July/ August 2006.

A tough choice

Just because new drugs arrive, we must not assume that *because* they're new, they're problem-free. There appears to be nothing that doesn't have implications for the rest of our health, unless we take a completely different route through medicine that is ecological and won't harm the body such as the ancient system of ayurvedic medicine, the Gerson Therapy and other methods, all of which have very many success stories. Yet the medical establishment refuses to accept any of these as a treatment for breast cancer or any other cancer. It is therefore not surprising that we can feel totally disempowered by the fact that, whether we like it or not, we are given no choice but to take such highly toxic, carcinogenic drugs.

Healthy prevention

At a preventative level, it is important to know that these patented drugs are not alone in locking into the body's oestrogen receptors. Soy and many other natural alternatives also work in the same way and are healthy phyto-oestrogens, the 'good' oestrogen as opposed to the 'bad', but not a great money-spinner for the pharmaceutical companies as they are natural products. Undoubtedly diet and supplements, the avoidance of environmental hazards, homeopathy and a host of natural therapies, can contribute greatly to the balance of oestrogens and other hormones and, as research shows, help towards preventing breast cancer.

Cause and prevention needed

It takes very little imagination to understand the dilemma all women face when trying to find the best way to be rid of breast cancer, whilst at the same time being confronted with this sort of conflicting information. As more women voice their concerns and some turn away from tamoxifen and similar drugs, the medical establishment and scientific researchers must understand the very clear message we are giving to them – that we consider this treatment is not only risky, but potentially highly damaging. Already, more than 30 years have been given to administering breast cancer drugs on a vast scale through our health services. We will be better served when the medical establishment acknowledges there are safer methods of diagnosis and treatment that can recognize possible causes, harmlessly instigate the potential reversal of the cancer and help provide effective prevention. This should be a priority. We have waited too long.

10 Other Women's Stories

The dream

Find me a woman who wouldn't want to dream of a caring GP telling her that, although she has breast cancer, it is a minor illness which can easily be dealt with, without surgery or any side effects from medication. All she has to do is follow a programme that will leave her in better health than before and she can be certain that neither she nor her family have any cause to worry. This is the dream that urgently needs to become a reality.

The present reality

Many readers may already be familiar with other women's stories as these are frequently published in newspapers, magazine articles and books. All the stories show the remarkable bravery of those women who have or have had breast cancer. Women of all ages – from the exceptionally young, to those much older – deal with their illness with courage and realism, whatever the course of treatment they may have chosen to take. Their stories speak for themselves.

One woman, when faced with a recurrence, decided that as the standard treatments had failed, she would try the Gerson Therapy. Gathering as much information as she could, she changed her diet and imported the recommended juicer from the USA. Up to this point her diet had been dominated by fast food, so it required her to make a huge change. She persisted with the new diet and became much healthier, but not completely clear of the cancer. Very much a career woman, in her forties, she thought that the best idea would be to go to Mexico, the home of the Gerson treatment. There she finally became free from cancer and for a few years remained in good health, until she chose to return to a highly stressful job and again began indulging her love of fast food, taking a cavalier 'I don't care, I'm all right now' attitude. Ultimately, the idea of a permanently healthier lifestyle proved too much for her, the cancer returned, and sadly she died.

Writer and producer Sarah Parkinson chose her own way through her dilemma with breast cancer. When she died, many paid tribute to Sarah and the inner strength she had shown throughout. I spoke with her a few times and it was clear that she had the most remarkable spirit and passion to live her life to the full. Sarah, wife of the television personality and entertainer Paul Merton, believed that her treatment with IVF had caused her breast cancer and refused chemotherapy believing she would not survive the harsh treatment. Sarah was the voice of so very many young women today, whose great fear on finding that they have breast cancer is that they may not be able to conceive as a consequence of the treatments.

Amanda Jones, 40, is one of many who say that the possibility of conceiving is almost non-existent because of the treatment she has received – surgery, chemotherapy and radiotherapy. For her, this is devastating. Like many women, she says that she still checks her breasts frequently each day. She has faced her problems with great bravery and has done everything she can to enhance the quality of her day-to-day life. She feels that alternative therapies, including Chinese medicine and homeopathy, have benefited her greatly.

Helen Howland, a stunningly beautiful woman, married with

two young children, refused further treatment of a mastectomy, chemotherapy and radiotherapy believing that these would be destructive to her. However, like me, Helen regained her health by choosing a complete regeneration treatment supported with complementary therapies. With her husband and children she moved away from the hectic pace of London city life to be near nature and the sea. Here she is living life to the full in the most extraordinarily vibrant and exemplary way.

There are many stories and plenty of evidence to be found of other women who have had breast cancer and regained their health with no further recurrence and without opting for surgery, chemotherapy or radiotherapy. There are plenty of scientific papers that speak out against these conventional cancer treatments and many others that ask why successful non-invasive treatments continue to be suppressed, but these are the ones we never hear about. If you have access to the Internet, a good introduction to these papers is the article 'Scientific Cancer Treatment?'[1]

Finding the most beneficial treatment for you

After serious contemplation, the most prudent course of action is to become informed and seek what you believe will be the best for you. Then, if you decide to take the conventional route believing that it will be beneficial, be fully empowered in the knowledge that this is the right choice for you. Whatever we choose, if we have every confidence in our choice then we actively enhance the possibility of a more satisfactory outcome.

I remember talking to a young woman in her thirties who was recovering from breast cancer and, like many women now, she had decided to have some of the conventional treatment, but not all of it. In addition she chose to use various complementary therapies which she believed were helping her through her treatment. It was a strain on her finances to pay for the complementary therapies, but she believed they were helping her enormously on her road back to health. This is a very common story these days, many women believing that complementary medicine in addition to conventional medicine can be greatly advantageous. It is not difficult to understand this personal choice as it would appear to be beneficial and offer protection from the harshness of conventional treatment. But although it may be successful for some, it may possibly become an unwitting compromise for others. In either case, it is essential to be under the guidance of a holistic doctor who understands and specializes in breast cancer. Having taken all these factors into account I decided that for me it would be preferable to take the orthodox regeneration treatment that I was offered in Germany.

The right to choose

There appears to be the beginning of a sea change in women's attitude to the treatment of breast cancer. I have become aware in the last two years of an increasingly large group of women, often young women, some single, others married or in partnerships, with or without children, who are not prepared to be coerced, and in some cases bullied, into taking steps with their own health which they feel could be damaging. These women value highly the quality of their lives and their families and are not happy to settle for what, in some cases, could be permanent damage as a result of the conventional treatments. Whatever other treatments they settle for, none of these women take their decisions lightly. Their lives are at stake. They know it is just possible that they might recover with conventional treatment, but they see it as an enormous risk and have a sound instinct that it is not the route that will best serve either their present or future health. I marvel at the way so many women diligently search out very complex information about breast cancer, once they are faced with the disease. Their knowledge of the various possible treatments for breast cancer can be astonishing, women often networking information between each other and giving each other tremendous support.

Each woman must choose the best for herself, whilst recognizing the need to discern between 'fear' and what simply 'feels wrong' when making these choices. The dignity of being allowed a choice in the way our bodies are treated, and what happens to them, is our fundamental right.

A Questionnaire

Whilst writing this book I decided to formulate a questionnaire of frequently *unasked* questions in order to get a better and broader understanding of the experiences of other women with breast cancer. I gave questionnaires to Breast Cancer Haven and also to those who requested them at a talk I gave to the Clouds Trust in 2003. A few of these women then passed the questionnaire on to others. Of the women who received the questionnaire, some never completed it: I sympathize with them as some were too immersed in trying to cope with current treatments, whilst others understandably had a problem recalling details which they were happier to forget. However, seven women, all from different backgrounds, patiently set to work to provide a valuable insight. I knew only one of the women beforehand, but I soon began to feel that I knew the others after receiving their returned questionnaires and reading their very poignant stories. In some cases women's names have been changed at their request.

The women, Maisie, Ann, Linda, Sylvia, Pat, Diana and Patricia, ranged in age from 44 to 61. They came from different parts of the UK: Middlesex, Hertfordshire, West Sussex, Derbyshire, Surrey and two from Aberdeen, Scotland. The woman that I already knew had been diagnosed in 1994, when she was told that she was 'precancerous'. She was the only one out of the seven who had found her treatment and those involved with it to be satisfactory. The other six were diagnosed between 2001 and 2004. Most of the women were treated by the NHS, just two were treated privately.

The questions and their answers are as follows, with the women's own words being reproduced as they were written on the questionnaire.

Did you discover you had cancer through self-examination, another person, doctor, mammogram, any other means?

1 Self-examination
2 Self-examination
3 Self-examination
4 Self-examination
5 Mammogram
6 Full medical examination
7 Mammogram

How did you feel physically and mentally just prior to being diagnosed?

1 V.V. Frightened and I passed out and couldn't understand what was happening. I asked why and was told that it did not matter – it now needed to be treated.
2 I had been feeling tired but otherwise absolutely fine.
3 Well physically. Very anxious mentally.
4 Anxious and afraid. Physically – fine.
5 Sick and sweaty, frightened like it was a dream.
6 Fine
7 [Not answered.]

When were you given the diagnosis, what did they tell you and how did you react?

1 2003. First diagnosis. I had to have a biopsy to ascertain what type of cancer (grade) then a lumpectomy and radiotherapy. After lumpectomy (well just before surgery) – told I would need another operation (i.e. mastectomy) chemotherapy and radiotherapy. Because of radiotherapy no reconstruction after the mastectomy.
2 November 2003. I was told the result of the needle biopsy was that cancerous cells were present in a lump.
3 July 2003. Told me it was cancer and then sent me for a biopsy. Already knew in myself what the diagnosis would be.

4 March 2001. 'It was bad news' – aggressive breast cancer. Burst into tears – shock – thought I was going to die very soon.

5 January 2004. You have breast cancer. Very calm and matter-of-fact. Tears came later!!

6 July 1994. On a scale of 1–5 (5 being cancer) – you are between 3 and 4, precancerous. Calmly, but in denial – tried to listen and understand what he was saying.

7 16 May 2002. [Remainder of question not answered.]

Did you ask for a second opinion?

1 Yes – I went to an anthroposophical German doctor who recommended I start Iscador (mistletoe) and gave me Jane Plant's book. I read [it] and I cut out dairy. V. HELPFUL – A LIFELINE.

2 No

3 No

4 No, but asked if they were sure.

5 Yes. But I got told off for asking and never got one anyway.

6 No

7 No

What treatment was recommended?

1 Oncologist said (after mastectomy) I must have chemotherapy.

2 A lumpectomy followed by radiotherapy and possibly chemotherapy.

3 Lumpectomy and radiotherapy.

4 Surgery followed by chemotherapy and radiotherapy.

5 Lumpectomy and radiotherapy or mastectomy.

6 Two operations: Biopsy and removal of some lymph gland for tests, lumpectomy, physiotherapy and 5 weeks radiotherapy.

7 Mastectomy, chemotherapy and radiotherapy.

Did your doctor offer details of evidence that was based on the success of the treatment, or statistical ratings? **[Only 2 of the 7 were offered the information.]**

1 I asked to see an oncologist. Only then was I told that chemotherapy was only 10% successful – or less – and that the chemotherapy could bring a 28% chance of heart damage, immunosuppression, baldness. All for only a 3–10% chance of help.

2 Yes

3 Yes

4 No

5 No

6 No

7 No. Only when I asked.

Were you offered or suggested any alternative treatment other than surgery, chemotherapy and radiotherapy – such as alternative or complementary therapies?

'No' for all seven women. One woman found other ways for herself after much searching.

At any time did you consider other options? If YES, what were they?

1 I refused chemo as I was told I had a 'poor prognosis' – I was too frightened by the side effects of heart damage, etc. If I only had a year, then I didn't want to be ill the whole time from the treatment.

2 No

3 [Not answered.]

4 No – except to research complementary help.

5 Yes – Doing nothing!

6 No – but if it were today, I would combine the conventional with healing and alternative.

7 Yes – but didn't know what.

If you chose a different option to conventional treatment, what was it and why did you choose it?

Six women left this question blank. Number 1 gave the only reply and she didn't answer the question as such, but was clearly trying to find her way by rooting out what she thought to be the cause of her cancer.

1 Because my breast cancer was caused by being prescribed the mini-pill for 15 years following a miscarriage (to regulate the cycle); it increased progestogin i.e. *synthetic* hormone, not natural progesterone. (Refer to John Lee's book *Natural Progesterone.*) My GP issued a 'yellow card' as he said this was my main risk factor.

Did you feel pressured to accept the treatment on offer?

1. Yes
2. No
3. No
4 Yes
5. Yes
6 Yes
7 Yes

Did you feel a need to commence treatment urgently because of feeling anxious or panicky?

1 Yes. I just wanted to get on with it at first – due to fear.
2 Yes
3 Yes
4 Yes
5 Yes
6 Yes, but not because I felt panicky – more from a practical point of view.
7 No

*If you agreed to conventional treatment how soon after
diagnosis did the treatment commence?*

1 5 weeks, Iscador – at once.

2 2 weeks

3 6 weeks

4 4 weeks

5 6 days!! 6 days after diagnosis I had mastectomy.

6 some weeks

7 N/A (opted out of doing the suggested CPB –
   mastectomy, chemotherapy and radiotherapy) took
   tamoxifen for a year.

*If your treatments included chemotherapy and radiotherapy,
did they induce symptoms of menopause? YES/NO or were
you post-menopausal? YES/NO*

1 N/A. Refused chemotherapy and radiotherapy and my
   breast cancer was a non-hormone sensitive type. No.

2 Yes. No.

3 Yes. –

4 Yes. No.

5 –. Yes.

6 No. No.

7 Yes with tamoxifen.

*Did you experience any side effects from the treatment?
YES/NO. If YES please give details.*

1 I refused after surgery – then went to look for other
   options.

2 Yes. Complete hair loss and terrible nausea with
   chemotherapy.

3 Yes. Nausea, fatigue. Hot flushes.

4 Yes. Violent vomiting throughout.

5 Yes. Tamoxifen is causing dreadful sweats.

6 No.

7 [Not answered, but answered on the previous question.]

Was your treatment private... NHS... self-financed...in a country other than UK...?

1 NHS first. Second private.
2 Private
3 NHS and Private.
4 NHS
5 NHS
6 Private
7 [Not answered.]

If you had surgery was it a lumpectomy...YES/NO or mastectomy...YES/NO?

1 Both. After 3 weeks from lumpectomy, had mastectomy. It was too much and a great ordeal. Then I had a wound infection – so back in hospital for 3rd time for emergency antibiotics.
2 Lumpectomy
3 Lumpectomy
4 Mastectomy
5 Mastectomy
6 Lumpectomy
7 Didn't do either

Did you have any reconstructive surgery at the same time as the lumpectomy/mastectomy? YES/NO

1 No – told I could not as I had to have radiotherapy which would deform a reconstruction.
2 Yes
3 No
4 Yes
5 No – it was never mentioned.
6 No
7 N/A

Were you given photographs to view of the surgeon's work, or offered any opportunity to meet another patient who had undergone similar surgery? [Interestingly, this was answered out of the context of reconstruction by 2 women.]

1 No. She was a 'neat' surgeon – but now I think only the lumpectomy should have been done, not the mastectomy also. [This answer is about the surgery, not a reconstruction.]

2 No

3 No

4 Yes

5 No

6 N/A

7 N/A

If you underwent reconstruction were you happy with the final appearance of your breast(s)? YES/NO If unhappy with the results state why.

2 Yes

4 Yes. Protruding of implant at front side of breast.

Was recovery from the reconstruction straightforward in terms of soreness, infection or discomfort? If not state why.

2 Yes

4 Yes – apart from not able to use arm normally for over a year. Needed physiotherapy.

How did the follow-on treatment affect you, both physically and emotionally?

1 N/A

2 Hair loss was the worst thing that I have ever encountered.

3 [Not answered.]

4 Wrecked my body. Destroyed mentally. Confidence lost.

Fearful of leaving own home.

5 I had a pain problem from 8 years ago – much worse after the mastectomy.

6 Emotionally it didn't affect me at all – I had much support – physically felt fine too.

7 N/A

How well did the oncology team support you? Good support...Average support...Poor support...No support...

1 Average – but inappropriate pressure to conform – if you don't it is 'dangerous' etc.

2 Good

3 Good

4 Nothing to compare with, so can't say.

5 Average

6 Good

7 N/A

Were breast care nurses present at your appointments? YES/NO Did you value their support? YES/NO

1 She was too much 'with the surgeon' – not for me as a breast cancer sufferer. When I refused chemo, she did not contact me again. She/they are breast surgeon's nurses or oncologist's nurses as much as for the patient who goes along the 'normal' route – but if you refuse chemotherapy and radiotherapy – they do not help you.

2 Yes – sometimes they were at my appointments. Yes.

3 Yes/Yes

4 No/No

5 Yes, but not my breast care nurse. Yes.

6 Yes/Yes

7 Yes/No

Were you given any dietary advice during consultations?
YES/NO

1 Took advice from my own complementary/
   anthroposophical doctor, not from NHS.

2 Yes

3 No

4 No

5 No

6 No

7 No

How did your family and friends support you? If you were
employed, did you receive financial and emotional support
from your personnel department and colleagues?

1 Best support from The Clouds Trust and other breast
   cancer sufferers and 'taking my own responsibility'. Some
   good friends could not speak to me. Others I thought of
   as acquaintances became friends.

2 Good support.

3 Good in all cases.

4 Family no support.

5 Good

6 Good

7 [Not answered.]

If your clinical treatment is complete what type of follow-up
or monitoring are you being offered by the oncology team?

1 Not complete. I have a new tumour (under one arm). But
   am dealing with it myself. I am using resonant
   frequencies and I think bio-physics will be future cancer
   treatment. If allowed into the mainstream.

2 Still having treatment.

3 6-monthly check-ups. Annual mammogram.

4 6-monthly check-ups.

5 I asked to see an oncologist and was told it was not
    necessary. Wanted to discuss my medication. Request
    refused.
6 Check-ups twice a year for 3 years and subsequently I
    have a mammogram and consultation each year.
7 N/A

**Do you feel the level of monitoring received is/was sufficient?
YES/NO If NO, what changes would make/have made you feel
more supported?**

1 I am against mammograms, as I think when I found the
    lump – the mammogram then 'squashed' the lump (it
    was very painful) and spread it to my lymph nodes.
2 Yes
3 Would have liked a body scan.
4 Yes, but any worries, I phone immediately to demand
    action.
5 It felt like I was on a conveyor belt from start to finish. No
    one had time to listen apart from family and friends.
6 Yes
7 N/A

**Is your view of the future optimistic, unchanged, anxious or
fearful?**

1 Optimistic
2 Optimistic
3 Optimistic
4 Optimistic
5 Fearful
6 Optimistic
7 [Not answered.]

Here are additional comments written by five of the seven women.

Maisie

I feel my hospital time – I had three stays, one for a lumpectomy operation, followed by another for a mastectomy and a stay because of a wound infection – *gave me time to think!* The small, wee voice at the back of my head argued that to take poisoning chemicals and radioactivity as a treatment is unacceptable. It is a gamble at best (10 per cent for chemotherapy and 25 per cent for radiotherapy) and for that low chance of success one risks 90 per cent worth of damage to the body including damaging the immune system which we need to fight the cancer.

I refused chemotherapy and radiotherapy (and now I wish I had refused surgery too – especially the mastectomy). As cancer is a metabolic disease, the tumour is merely acting as a 'thermometer'. What I did/am doing:

> Aug/Sept 03: Ukraine treatment and high dose vitamin C infusions (15 days at a clinic).
> Nov 03/Jan 04: Dendritic cell therapy (at a clinic).
> Apr 04/May 04: Started using Resonant Frequency (via Canadian company) and I notice my tumour is shrinking – so wish me luck!

Ann

Six months on from diagnosis. When I was told I had cancer, it was the most devastating thing that had happened to me since the death of my mother eight years previously. I was certainly in denial for about a month – 'this wasn't me – this was someone else – I had always been so healthy eh, eh.'

At the time, the consultant told me that eventually I might find that I gained from the whole experience and actually he was right. I have found an inner strength I never knew I had. I have found qualities in friends I never knew they had, and have found some friends perhaps were not what I thought they were.

It has been a big wake-up call for me and made me realize just how precious life is. My family and friends are so important to me and really, nothing else matters.

I'm hoping I may have become a better person through coping with this nightmare!

Good luck with the book.

Pat

I am most concerned that because of the area I live in (postcode lottery) I am not getting the best treatment in terms of medication. My worries and concerns were made light of, and I didn't feel I was getting the best from the consultant, the Breast Care Team and the hospital. The only real support I have had (apart from friends and family who have been wonderful) has been from The London Haven [now renamed Breast Cancer Haven].

I wish I lived in an area where I could get the best!!

Diana

Having been delivered my scenario, I was actually offered counselling immediately with a very experienced, sweet woman. As it happened I declined, but for someone else this could have been exactly what they needed if it was readily available.

Patricia

Around December 2001 I used to wake up thinking/working out how many people around me had breast cancer and what percentage I was in among friends and family. Something within me was saying I was in that percentage?

Had an ache under my right arm, thought it was bra wire.

> March 2002 – nipple had sunk in slightly.
> May 2002 – visit to doctors. I was sent for mammogram.
>   Bio. done following week. Four days later results.
> Route offered. Chemotherapy with 24-hour drip and three-
>   weekly, usual chemo.
> Checked out makes of chemo and effect on body.
> Asked oncologist what chances of permanent damage to

vital organs. He changed drug prescription without
saying a word.

Alarm bells rang!

Anyhow cancelled 1st July for 1st dose. Didn't go down
very well with doctors.

I was afraid of the chemo. Not the cancer.

The cancer has and does not bother me at all.

My diet got changed, my way of life changed too.

I have time that is mine 24/7 now.

Have learnt a lot and still learning today on alternatives.

Summary

All the women were told in a matter-of-fact way that they had cancer and in most cases a second opinion was not sought, one woman being 'told off' for asking for one. The only treatment available was surgery, chemotherapy and radiotherapy and usually tamoxifen as well. Just two of the seven were offered the success rate figures for the treatment and one who asked was given bleak statistics and a list of possible permanently damaging effects.

On considering their options, the one who was told of its damaging effects refused chemotherapy and researched other ways; one researched complementary methods; one said she thought of doing nothing; another wanted to do something else, but didn't know what. Two didn't consider anything else and one didn't answer the question. In the end, none took an alternative route, but several decided not to take the full treatment that had been prescribed.

Five out of seven felt pressured to start treatment and six of the seven felt they needed to start it urgently. The commencement of treatment varied from six days to six weeks after diagnosis. Tamoxifen produced hot flushes, and all the women who had chemotherapy developed menopausal symptoms. Violent vomiting, baldness, nausea, dreadful hot flushes and fatigue were reported. The surgeon's work was viewed by one of the two women who had opted for immediate reconstruction. One woman was satisfied with the result of the surgery and the other, although she indicated she was satisfied, then went on to list ongoing problems arising from the surgery.

By the time the question of follow-on treatment was reached, two women had opted out of the treatment, the precancerous one felt fine, one didn't answer and the other three who had taken further treatment reported severe pain problems, lost confidence, a wrecked body, being destroyed mentally and fearful of leaving home, with one finding that losing her hair was the worst thing she had ever encountered. Despite this list, three said the oncology support was good, two said it was average and another commented that she had nothing to compare it with. The valued support of breast care nurses and their attendance at the women's appointments was more or less satisfactory, but there was a feeling that these nurses were not always 'with or for them'.

Regarding diet, only one was given any advice. The support from outside, friends, colleagues and family was generally quite good, although one found her family of no help to her and another commented that some good friends were unable to speak to her, whilst acquaintances later became good friends.

Although one woman was still being treated and another had opted out, follow-up and monitoring left queries for several of the others. One, in retrospect, objected to mammograms, feeling them to be unsafe, one asked to see an oncologist and discuss medication and was refused; two women, who had finished their treatment, are being given annual mammograms.

Conclusion

My conclusions, borne out by the seven women and several others that I have spoken to, are highly consistent. It is quite clear that most women would prefer a different treatment to surgery, chemotherapy, radiotherapy and tamoxifen or similar drugs, but don't know what else to do as nothing else is offered. The result of this is that many women are only taking a part of the recommended treatment, a decision often based on readily available scientific evidence which they seek out themselves, along with an instinct for self-protection and survival. The main factors affecting their decision-making were doctors who have a holistic, sensitive and caring approach, other women, their experiences by word of mouth, and literature written by men and women who have researched other routes, plus sound common sense. Other women who opt out of the present treatment completely find that they are generally cast aside as being perverse, weird or uncooperative, being ostracized by the medical establishment and frequently refused help. In these circumstances they are left to their own devices to seek other treatments at their own expense.

Clearly the vast majority of women feel pressurized to begin their treatment immediately, and most receive considerable, bad and damaging side effects from the treatment. After the initial diagnosis a woman is often hastily put into the process without any idea of how she will look after surgery, something that is particularly important for those who have a reconstruction at the same time. Given the option, all the women that I have spoken to would prefer to see a woman who has actually had a reconstruction rather than a picture, and many don't even get to see a picture. As mentioned earlier in the book, the quality of the reconstruction is often a matter of luck, depending on where you live.

In spite of evidence concerning the association of diet with breast cancer, advice is not available except in rare cases, and, as we know, there is no prevention programme or detailed information available on the causes of breast cancer. The quality of follow-up appointments is mixed and, following breast cancer treatment, the previously infrequent monitoring by mammogram now becomes an annual event, with many women feeling distrustful of this form of screening.

The positive power of men and women

The grit and determination of women with breast cancer is remarkable. I marvelled at the bravery and enormous optimism of those women answering the questionnaire, despite their mostly difficult journeys. Whether they have breast cancer or not, patients can very often feel 'put down' by the cold, brusque attitude of a doctor. If we do have breast cancer, it is easy to see how such an attitude can undermine our confidence and leave us in a state of confusion and self-doubt.

Early in 2005, I read a most apposite interview with the actress Juliette Stevenson who was speaking about the extraordinary lack of women directors in the film industry, and giving a possible reason why this should be so. She said, 'Women entertain self-doubt more frequently than men do, and they are often good at self-parody.' How very true!

This shrewd observation is entirely in accord with my original and ongoing feeling that at the heart of the breast cancer problem and the unsatisfactory way in which it is currently being treated lies a general belief that the medical establishment knows best. Although many women may experience considerable doubts about the treatments they are given, generally they suppress these doubts – even to the point of making a joke about their condition – at the same time giving deference to the medical establishment. It is for these reasons that we so badly need the help and support of those scientists working without a vested interest in the pharmaceutical industry and the good men and women in our lives, to support us in what is tantamount to a battle to bring about the necessary but long overdue changes.

11 Politics

*The diseased empiricist mind is still ticking away
in its clock-like discreetness within the Newtonian
paradigm, oblivious of the holistic nature of all
reality.*

Henryk Skolimowski PhD, Professor of Philosophy,
Department of Humanities, University of Michigan.

Cancer research

When we consider the huge technological advances that have been
made in recent decades in so many fields affecting our daily lives,
how is it that the most widely advocated treatment for breast cancer
– surgery, chemotherapy and radiotherapy – is still in existence?
Surgery goes back hundreds of years whilst radiotherapy has been
used for approximately 100 years and chemotherapy for over 60
years. Even during the early days of chemotherapy there were
doubts amongst doctors about the importance that was being
attached to it. It is true that better, less brutal forms of treatment
exist, but these are not available in our present health care system.
Across the world there is much common ground in the understanding of cancer, so what exactly is cancer research doing? It
brings into question how, in the 21st century, we can still be no

nearer to *curing* breast cancer and many other cancers, when successful treatments are to be found, and quite clearly *have* been found in the past?

Looking at the World Cancer Research Fund (WCRF) website in 2004, I found under 'research' that it opened with:

> Science has only just begun to explore the relationships between what we eat, how we live and our risk of cancer. Expanding such knowledge is part of the World Cancer Research Fund's dual mission. For more than 20 years members of WCRF global network have fostered innovative research into the diet-cancer link providing the initial funding for many seminal projects. The world WCRF global network has drawn new scientists to the field and attracted additional funds from other sources for this important work. To date WCRF UK's research grant programmes have:
>
> • Provided more than £5 million in research funding.
>
> • Awarded over 55 research grants.
>
> • Provided research funding for more than 100 scientists working in 17 countries throughout the world ... [1]

Continuing in the section 'Expert Report' (Food, Nutrition and the Prevention of Cancer: A Global Perspective), we find that in 1993 the WCRF and the American Institute of Cancer Research (AICR) brought 16 experts together to:

> ... review scientific literature pertaining to the causal link between diet and cancer. In the previous decade thousands of research projects in this area had been conducted and reported in hundreds of scientific journals. The time had come to evaluate the evidence and ascertain what eating and exercise patterns are most likely

to influence the development of cancer ... The panel
reviewed more than 4,500 of the most recent and reliable
epidemiological, clinical and laboratory studies. The
review took three years and eventually involved more
than 100 scientists from around the world ... [2]

The above information was taken from the WCRF website on 15
March 2004, so I was naturally very surprised to find another
website which, a *month earlier* had been quite clear and informative
about the possible causes of cancer. This second website was run by
The Cancer Prevention Research Trust UK, who appear to be
extraordinarily aware of the causes of cancer, and yet the only way
to find the relevant information is to scour the cancer websites. It is
not the sort of information that comes readily to the public's
attention:

One in three of all persons born in the United Kingdom
develops some form of cancer during his or her lifetime
... Cancer is not one disease. It is a hundred or more
diseases. It can be induced in experimental animals by the
use of chemicals, radiations and viruses. Inspired by the
success of antibiotics in controlling infectious diseases,
the public, and indeed cancer research scientists have
been concentrating in seeking a cure. It is just possible
that for many of the forms of cancer there will be no
magic cure and the most practical approach will be to
find a means of prevention and prophylaxis ... Many
specialists in the field of cancer research now believe that
chemicals present in food and the environment in general
are responsible for 80–90% of all cancer in humans; the
remainder are believed to be caused by radiation or
viruses. Current evidence suggests that there exists no
safe threshold level for a carcinogenic chemical. [3]

So what is being done about it? It is not difficult to imagine that somewhere in the field of cancer research, scientists might be tempted to throw their hands in the air and say, 'It's all too complicated,' and stay within the more easily manageable parameter of searching for a 'cure'.

In October 2000, Martin J Walker wrote an article entitled 'Your Money and Your Life' for the *Ecologist* magazine revealing exactly what goes on in the money-spinning cancer industry. He pointed out that the UK had over 600 cancer charities, which by 2004 had risen to 650. I recommend anyone to read the full article, but here are some extracts:

> Britain's cancer charities are a multi-million pound industry. But they are no nearer to 'curing' cancer than they were half a century ago. Quite the opposite – much of their time and money is spent avoiding awkward questions about what causes the disease. The cancer establishment's refusal to research environmental and chemical causes of cancer could, perhaps, be seen as a sin of crude omission. But its determined and continual assault on all and any 'alternative' therapies and practitioners reveals the charities in their true colours – as footsoldiers for the chemical industry and the conventional medical establishment.
>
> The high point of scientific medicine's assault upon alternative approaches to cancer was the 1939 Cancer Act, which coincidentally came into being in the same year that the International Cancer Research Fund (ICRF) was granted a Royal Charter and Charitable Status. The act forbade, on pain of draconian punishment, anyone other than a qualified doctor, involved in work with cancer, from speaking about the causes or the treatment of cancer. From that point on, the cancer establishment and its partners in industry launched an all-out war on alternative approaches to cancer, which is still being fought today.

When asked about funding, the bigger charities point to their fundraising pie charts, which show that their major funding comes in individual covenants and donations, with only relatively minor amounts given by corporate sponsors. Yet this is to miss the point; for the big cancer research charities are steeped in an industrial culture which can serve to hide serious conflicts between the need for preventative research and the needs of the industry. Both the Cancer Research Campaign (CRC) and the ICRF hold substantial reserves – in the mid 90s the ICRF's tied assets stood at £90m – most of which is invested in industry. Even as late as the mid 90s it was revealed that the ICRF was 'inadvertently' investing in the tobacco industry. The investment portfolio of the cancer charities is not publicly accessible, and consequently it is not possible for supporters to ensure that investments have only been made in companies which are not implicit in the production of carcinogens.

Apart from the continual propaganda about cigarettes, there is no public discourse about the chemical or environmental causes of cancer. And it is unlikely that the public will ever be informed about them while cancer research in Britain is dominated by a cabal of unaccountable doctors, scientists and surgeons – a 'cancer club' which garners some of its funding and much of its philosophy from an industrial infrastructure which independent scientists believe is itself the cause of rising cancer rates. As science and medicine have become increasingly interlocked with industry, the motivation, initiative and funding for preventative cancer research has all but dried up. The conclusion today is inescapable: Britain's cancer research charities are part of the problem, not the solution.

The big cancer charities' effective monopoly is

unaccountable to the people who fund them with
voluntary contributions or the representatives of those
who leave them bequests. Although they dictate NHS
policy on cancer, they are unaccountable to parliament or
the public. The power and independence of the cancer
charities owe a lot to the continuing unwillingness of
government to become involved financially and
scientifically in cancer research. Only by removing the
dependency of cancer researchers on private money can
research become honest again.

Office-holders and scientists working in cancer
research should have to make a public declaration of all
their interests in pharmaceutical or biotech companies.
These declarations, together with staff salary figures,
should be made publicly available. All cancer research
scientists should also have to spend a major part of their
time on non-chemical, non-genetic treatments or
environmental causes of cancer. [4]

The Cancer Prevention Research Trust states that its sacred mission
is the prevention of cancer. In the June 2006 edition of its
newsletter *Cancer Prevention And Health News*, it points out that
cancer treatments increase the risk of further cancers, nerve
damage, other illnesses and stroke in later life and that chemotherapy can damage the peripheral and the central nervous system
with resulting weakness, numbness and pain in the extremities,
impaired cognition, loss of memory and loss of sight. Children
treated with radiotherapy for some diseases have a much greater
chance of strokes. If you continue reading, you certainly would
object strongly to being given these treatments. But what are organizations such as the World Cancer Research Fund, or our health
authorities doing about it? Where is the prevention? Why haven't
these drugs been banned?

Medical editor Lois Rogers wrote an article under the headline
'Cancer cases will treble in a generation, warn doctors' in the

Sunday Times of 13 June 2004. The article was a product of a think tank funded by the Macmillan Cancer Relief charity, highlighting the dangers of a lack of long-term health care planning by government and the potential bankrupting of the NHS because of the expensive treatments cancer patients require. It pointed out that instead of funding prevention, 98 per cent of research is into lucrative drugs for treatments, most of these holding out the false promises of cure. Consider the phenomenal cost of drugs to the NHS each year; it is estimated that the annual budget is likely to reach £90 billion by 2007.

Does the person who sets out to raise funds for cancer research charities really understand what happens to the money they collect, out of their goodwill to assist in eradicating cancer? How well informed are we about how this money will be used? Do they believe a 'cure' is just around the corner? This doesn't appear to be the case. Perhaps we should ask how much scrutiny is given to the new so-called wonder drugs.

How we are affected

In an article entitled 'How Scientific Are Orthodox Cancer Treatments?' Walter Last, the biochemist and science and health writer wrote:

> In 1993, the editor of *The Lancet* pointed out that, despite various modifications of breast cancer treatment, death rates remained unchanged. He acknowledged that despite the almost weekly releases of miracle breakthroughs, the medical profession with its extraordinary capacity for self-delusion (his words, not mine) in all truth has lost its way. At the same time he rejected the view of those who believe that salvation will come from increasing chemotherapy after surgery to just below the rate where it kills the patient. He asked, 'Would it not be more scientific to ask why our approach has failed?' Not too

soon to ask this question after a century of mutilating women, I would say. The title of this editorial appropriately, is 'Breast cancer, have we lost our way?'

After an analysis of several large mammogram screening studies found that mammography leads to more aggressive treatment with no survival benefits, even the editor of *The Lancet* had to admit that there is no reliable evidence from large randomized trials to support mammography screening programs. The significance of this statement goes far beyond the use of mammograms.

Research studies and unbiased statistical analysis show that there is no scientific basis for orthodox cancer treatments like radical surgery, chemotherapy and radiation therapy and that these treatments often do more harm than good. Researchers have said it is complacent to continue subjecting at least 70% of women with breast cancer to a futile mutilating procedure. Furthermore, there is no evidence that early mastectomy affects survival; if patients knew this, they would most likely refuse surgery.

In cancer research, success – expressed as a five-year survival rate – is established by comparing other forms and combinations of treatment with the results from surgery alone. However, the success rate of surgery has rarely been compared with the survival rates of untreated patients and never with patients who adopted natural therapies. Therefore orthodox cancer treatment is basically unscientific. The overall supposed cure rate is not higher than can be accounted for by spontaneous remissions and the placebo effect.

Common ways to make medical statistics look more favourable are as follows. Patients who die during prolonged medical treatment with chemotherapy or radiotherapy are not counted in the statistics because they did not receive the full treatment. In the control group, everyone who dies is counted. Furthermore, success commonly is judged by the percentage of shrinking tumours, regardless of patient survival; but if the rate or length of survival is measured, then it is usually only in terms of dying from the treated disease. It is not normally shown how many of the patients die due to the treatment itself. [5]

Massive fatalities occur through drugs and yet, dismissing the wishes of the population it represents, the UK government condones the European Union (EU) restrictions on vitamin and other supplements, preferring to support the pharmaceutical companies who supply prescribed drugs and toxic treatments. Referring to the editorial 'Death by Medicine' by Richard Smith in the *British Medical Journal* Walter Last says:

Yet only 15% of medical interventions are supported by scientific evidence ... This is because only 1% of the articles in medical journals are scientifically sound, and partly because many treatments have never been assessed at all. [6]

Walter Last quotes Ulrich Abel, the respected German biostatistician who stated that 'Many oncologists take it for granted that response to therapy prolongs survival, an opinion which is based on fallacy and which is not supported by clinical studies.' Walter Last's article in *Nexus Magazine* continues:

Despite a majority of Western populations preferring natural remedies, basically all political parties promote dependency on pharmaceutical drugs. Therefore as a first step to changing this oppressive political climate, we urgently need a political party that promotes natural health care rather than drug dependency ...

> Would it not be more scientific to evaluate the
> methods of natural cancer therapists impartially rather
> than put the therapists in jail? Most alternative cancer
> clinics in the USA have had to relocate to Mexico. (For a
> list of such clinics see the website
> http://www.cancercure.org) ... Many natural cancer
> therapists claim a success rate of more than 90% in
> arresting and reversing cancer, provided that patients
> have not been subjected to orthodox treatments
> beforehand. The most damaging treatments appear to be
> chemotherapy and radiotherapy. [7]

The question is, just how damaging? Conventional chemotherapy agents are classified as 'cytotoxic' so just *how* toxic are these chemotherapy drugs? I suggest you arm yourself with a tin hat and a cup of tea before continuing.

It appears that chemotherapy units in hospitals regard accidents with chemotherapy drugs as highly hazardous. If there is an accident with these chemical agents, there must be a health and safety plan providing controls and policies for clearing up such chemical spills. Some of these plans may even suggest preventing exposure by finding safer alternatives if possible, as some of these chemical agents can cause burning if they touch the body. Should a spill greater than a teaspoon occur, it is likely that a hazard team may need to be called in. If the problem is smaller, then it can be dealt with by cordoning off the area and putting on a fully protective overall, covers for footwear, goggles, protective gloves and a mask. After cleaning up with special substances and materials, the procedure for disposing of the contaminated waste requires strict adherence with several plastic bags being utilized and then placed inside further plastic bags.

Overkill in general

Overkill has always been a problem in any situation, whether globally or individually. Wars are perhaps the best example, where annihilation of the enemy with weaponry which is highly dangerous to those using it, as well as to those it targets, has been used to extreme, causing the most appalling loss of innocent lives. At an individual level, avoiding overkill comes naturally to most of us on a daily basis – we are well aware of the problems it can cause. It is detrimental when it applies to the teaching of children where a rigid, fanatical approach is taken: it causes fear, frustration and insecurity. Likewise, musicians who are hell-bent on achieving the world's best technique can cause themselves physical injury whilst at the same time stunting their interpretive growth and powers. Wherever and however we meet with excess, Mother Nature has a way of redressing the balance.

The media

In the public arena, the media provide material fed from the political hothouse of cancer, and are responsible for bringing us as clear and truthful a picture as possible. Television, Ceefax, newspapers and magazines drip feed us information at remarkably regular intervals – usually every two weeks – about an 'exciting new breakthrough in cancer'. I have come to the conclusion that this is a placebo sent out to the nation to keep us buoyant and hopeful. Often the 'news' is simply 'old news' recycled. Christmas is a time when we are guaranteed to be given glad tidings, presumably to make our Yuletide brighter. In 2004, the news was about the breast cancer drug Arimidex, but this had already been the 'news' of Christmas 2001 (*see* page 43). If we observe carefully, it is easy to see not only these 'coincidences', but also journalists reporting hard facts in such a way that we do not feel alarmed, bringing the reader to the point of being able to dismiss as 'not very important', facts that are deeply disturbing.

In February 2004, the *Sunday Times Style Magazine* ran an article entitled 'Deodorant: The Truth' by Sally Brown; a strange piece which posed more questions than it answered. Commenting on the research of Dr Philippa Darbre, Senior Lecturer in Oncology at the University of Reading, into the connection of deodorant use and breast cancer, research chemist Dr Stephen Antczak contradicted Dr Darbre by saying, 'There is compelling evidence that antiperspirants do not contribute to breast cancer'. However, he gave no evidence in the article to support his statement and, apparently, the evidence is not to be found. Dr Darbre, a leading figure internationally in this field of research, reveals that at the time of this article there was a grand total of two papers in the database, the first in 2002 which was inconclusive and another in 2003 showing that those with breast cancer who had used deodorant and antiperspirant products had an earlier age of diagnosis of breast cancer by up to 22 years. She stresses the urgent need for more primary scientific research. None of this information was used in the *Sunday Times* article. However the story did not end there.

Dr Darbre had analyzed tumours removed from women *before* they received further treatment, and discovered that these tumours contained the chemical parabens found in deodorants. Dr Antczak went on to say, 'Frankly we would be surprised if parabens were not found in the tumours, because many of the drugs used to treat cancers contain parabens, and these drugs may well have been directly injected into the tumours or the tumour cells.' At this point I had to reread the article to see if I had been asleep, as Dr Antczak's comments sounded completely wrong. From my research, I believed that Dr Darbre had done the tests on women who had *not* been exposed to anti-cancer drugs prior to the tumour analysis and indeed this proved to be the case when I asked Dr Darbre. [8]

The article brought two major breast cancer issues to our attention, firstly that parabens are highly dangerous in the carcinogenic picture. Secondly, Dr Antczak made it quite clear that anti-cancer drugs actually contain parabens – this appalling fact only emerging, seemingly, by chance. To many people it will be an astonishing revelation that cancer is being treated with carcinogenic drugs. Because of the strange way in which the article was written, the reader would very likely have missed this second point, the whole piece leaving them with a dubious and mixed message which appeared to imply 'we don't want to scare you'. Is this one of the main reasons why we are frequently not told the truth? The breast cancer charities and, of course, the Toiletry and Perfume Association, seemed to be quick to play down any problems with these products, but that is the way these bodies tend to communicate with us; above all, they don't want to rock the boat or, most importantly, upset sales.

Corporate giants

Research chemists who work for chemical, pesticide, pharmaceutical and toiletry companies have an agenda to produce research evidence to counter claims that their products are unsafe or that they put users at risk. Also, the financial muscle of these corporate giants means that they have sufficient money to fund legal actions to quell opposition. My interpretation is that this industry appears to be driven by finance and politics rather than health. But unless health is the principal driving force, it is almost inevitable that medical research programmes will be compromised. The extent to which genuine research has already been compromised is illustrated in the article 'Scientific Cancer Treatment?', which reports that US Senators were so impressed with the results of Dr Gerson's cancer therapy that a Senate Committee 'moved strongly to provide extensive funds for research' into the treatment. But, the report continues, '… the American Medical Association lobbied so strongly against research into nutritional cancer therapies that the move was defeated in the Senate, although only by four votes.' [9]

The lack of prevention in the community

We have no prevention programme for breast cancer currently available, which is not surprising as it is not seen to be the most important issue, with so little time and money given to prevention research. Consequently, if you are concerned about cancer prevention – as so many women are – there is no knowing whether or not your GP would be helpful in giving preventative advice, unless he or she happens to have a particular interest in breast cancer. In his address to a public meeting held on 17 March 2001 in Boston, England, entitled 'Working in partnership with healthcare professionals' and organized by Lincolnshire Against Cancer, Women's Environmental Network and PEX, Professor Andrew Watterson stated:

> There have been accusations that communities cry wolf. But at the centre of the NHS health plans for Scotland, England and Wales there is the intention of involving patients and communities. If people say they are concerned about cancer, you would have thought that healthcare professionals would welcome them with open arms. But their response is not to have an informed debate but simply to dismiss them.

Mechanical medicine

Criticism of the medical establishment runs high in many quarters. Listening to women who have had breast cancer and those who have had to care for, or provide some kind of service to breast cancer patients, it is clear that most of those involved regard the process as lacking, and regard the first port of call – the surgeon – as a mechanic who often shows a noticeable lack of personal communication and feeling.

For many of us, the word 'mechanic' brings to mind a car in the garage for repair. We deliver the car to the garage and then leave it entirely in the hands of the mechanics, knowing that they have learnt through instruction how to deal with such problems. It helps if they have had some reasonable amount of experience, so when you tell them what's wrong, the chances are they will have come across the problem before with an identical or similar model, therefore making the whole procedure of diagnosis and repair much more straightforward. If you have been treated for breast cancer, this approach will sound familiar.

The dictionary defines 'mechanic' as, 'Pertaining to or involving manual labour or skill. Of the nature of or pertaining to a machine or machines; worked by machinery. Worked or working like a machine; acting mechanically...involuntary, automatic. Pertaining to, produced by, or dominated by physical forces. Interpreting and explaining the phenomena of the universe by reference to causally determined material forces; mechanistic.' [10]

Mechanical performances

For me, the most poignant description of the plural of the noun 'mechanic' is: 'the technical or procedural aspects of something; "grasps the mechanics of music but has no feel for it".'[11] As a professional musician, however good a technician you are, it is well nigh impossible to make a successful career, unless you have the 'feel' – meaning in this case, spirit, mind and psychology. Fortunately, the public tend to be very discerning when it comes to hearing 'the real thing' – the truly consummate performance. However, where science and medicine are concerned the public's opinion is more or less completely ignored. Instead, those who work in these two fields appear to be subject exclusively to peer review.

As an artist, you are judged to be only as good as your last performance. Much like a football or tennis player, a musician performing live is totally transparent for all to see. Those who recognize a poor performance in any of these activities are at liberty to walk away at any time. Bearing this in mind, perhaps we should consider walking away and following some other path for our breast cancer treatment.

Diagnostic machinery

It is not only many surgeons who take a mechanistic approach. As science has progressed, an ever growing number of increasingly sophisticated mechanical devices is being used to 'look' at our bodies in the hope of getting a greater understanding of our illnesses.

Writing in 2003, Bill Sturgeon pointed to the potential problems related to diagnostic machinery:

> The 'machinery' of the laboratory where cancer is diagnosed is also a problem. Irwin D. Bross, PhD, former director of bio-statistics at the Roswell Park Memorial Cancer Hospital, America, discovered over half of the breast cancer diagnoses had benign lesions that were unable to spread. He said that under a light microscope, they look like cancer. He also pointed out that as the function of the sex organs diminishes, breast cancer and prostate cancer can show cells which often become abnormal, but are not cancerous.[12]

Present performance and integrity

In January 2005, the Public Accounts Committee of the House of Commons announced that England, Scotland and Wales were lagging far behind most of Western Europe in its cancer survival rates, with the likelihood of people dying from cancer in the North of England being twice that of those in the South. In many cases they found delays in treatment and a lack of available drugs. France has the best survival rates for breast cancer, followed closely by other major European countries. Will this alarming information bring about the urgently needed changes in the UK, or will it be brushed aside?

Body factories

Mechanics and machines belong in a sterile, purely functional environment, not a place of comfort. Sadly, many hospitals fit this description. Being married to an architect who is sensitive to the built environment and the needs of those living, working and playing in it, I recognize the subtleties that pervade his world when comparing it to my world of music – subtleties that stretch way beyond mere technicalities. Whatever our field of specialization, we still need to remain sensitive to the bigger picture. Plato recognized the need for an all-embracing education where, for example, architects, musicians and doctors were required to have a knowledge and understanding of many subjects, otherwise they were not considered adequate to be in their profession.

Living in north London, I have seen the new University College Hospital grow from the roots. There for the world to see, it stands on the pavement of the very busy Euston Road, bordering Gower Street and Tottenham Court Road. It is enormous. The building is a construction of green-coloured glass, cold and dominant, and I would prefer not to have to be ill in there simply because it looks so austere. As Tom and I once drove past the almost completed building, I remarked that it looked like a body factory, and wondered why it had to be like this. Imposing itself on the landscape, no doubt the NHS were duly impressed that it looked so powerful, but is this what we really want? The government in its obsession with 'targets' and 'increased productivity' has created a health service run by managers and bureaucrats who work from the hospitals. Perhaps this is why these buildings look so austere. Would it not be preferable to create a hospital which first and foremost considers the patient and his or her needs, making the environment more welcoming and nurturing to both body and spirit? What we have at present is stark and functional, the patient having to fit in with the hospital agenda rather than the other way around. It cannot be easy in these circumstances to create healthy, caring relationships between medical staff and patients. But the implications of such buildings go much further. In his book, *The Boiled Frog Syndrome*, Thomas Saunders tells us:

> The continuous bright general lighting conditions usually found in hospitals were linked to a number of health problems in animals and humans, including retinal pathology, disruption of circadian rhythms, reduced melatonin secretion, sleeplessness, fatigue, cognitive difficulties and behavioural patterns.[13]

In the case of infants, it appears that when these problems are eradicated, they return to a normal growth and development pattern, with reduced stress levels. Surely the last thing we want in our hospitals is increased stress and dis-ease, we *need* to feel that the hospital is a place of nurture and beauty as well as being a place where we receive treatment, where our spirits can be uplifted and above all, where we can begin to be healthy again.

Professor Henryk Skolimowski revealed that Hippocrates and the ancient Greeks had a much greater understanding of our needs:

> The Esclapeion was a place of healing as well as a place of learning of medicine, a combined medical academy and a hospital, or a university hospital. Some 6,000 medical herbs were recognized and used. The knowledge of the organism and its reactions to herbs must have been gloriously studied … While our medical centres are places of sterility, places which we want to leave as soon as possible, it was quite the opposite with the esclepia of Ancient Greece … Situated in inspiring surroundings, sheltered by classical buildings and temples, an esclapeion was a place you wanted to stay, not to leave as soon as possible. The healing surrounding the place was one of its primary assets. You can still feel it, after twenty-four centuries of destruction, when you find yourself at Epidaurus, at Delphi or at the esclapeion of Kos.[14]

Minus the politics

Whilst those who create the hospitals follow their dream of how a hospital should look in the 21st century, it might be better to start to think about how it must feel to be ill and begin to plan for the patient's need to become whole and healthy. If the medical establishment continues to condone those areas of our health care that lack integrity, from breast cancer treatments to the buildings that they create, nothing will change. It requires them to make a stand. Health care workers are functioning in a flawed system for their training is confined to a pharmaceutical-based health service which, as a consequence, perpetuates its own problems through the narrowness of its vision. There must be many doctors and nurses who feel desperately compromised in their attempts to treat 'the whole person'. Mainstream medicine leaves no room for this approach, requiring them to put their philosophy, belief and integrity second to the government, the pharmaceutical industry, large amounts of administration and shortages of both staff and time. General practitioners are no longer empowered and the system they work in does not seem aware of the evidence that only 12.5 per cent of illness is biological. It is thought that a further 50 per cent is due to social problems, 25 per cent to psychological and 12.5 per cent to psychosomatic problems. Not only are doctors driven by endless red tape, but in the UK they have to act as social carers thanks to our well-evolved 'nanny state'. This, plus the powerful pressure of the pharmaceutical industry turns the doctor's job into one of frustration and compromise, the system taking priority over the patient. To deal properly with those who are ill, doctors need time and sensitivity: the present system leaves no room for either.

In medicine, the political act of pleasing bureaucracy within bureaucracy appears to have become a huge problem. Here I am referring to those bodies that are given official government approval and which begin their enquiries by outsourcing to find the truth and efficacy of specific research, only to end up with endless working parties and a statement which – often by omission of data – is more in the nature of a watered down half-truth. This leaves not only those passionately involved in the search for truth for the benefit of humanity, but humanity itself, yet again, compromised.

Surely, at best we would all want to pursue that which is beautiful, positive, informed and in the light; all things which are stripped of half-truths, compromise and uncertainty. In this situation body, mind, emotions and spirit work in synchronicity in order to attain that which is beneficial to us all. This attitude needs to apply to medicine as much as to music, literature, architecture, art, science, industry and the world in general, if we are to be whole, and protected from discord in our bodies and lives.

PART THREE

Getting To The Heart Of Cancer

If you want to understand what something is, you must look and see where it came from.

Goethe

The cure of the part should not be attempted without the treatment of the whole.

Plato

I will apply dietetic measures for the benefit of the sick ...

The Hippocratic Oath
Classical version, translated by Louis Edelstein 1943
(No longer used in the modern version)

12 The Golden Key – A Systemic Disease

'Systemic' (siste-mik) … Physiological and pathological: Belonging to, supplying, or affecting the system or body as a whole.

The Shorter Oxford English Dictionary

In a time when there is an urgent need to produce a therapy for cancer and no 'magic bullet' cure is available (and may never be), it would seem reasonable to expect research to investigate all possibilities, use all resources and efficiently pool information to address this complicated issue. Because the number of people with cancer is growing rapidly, it would be logical to follow up the work of those who are currently having success in treating cancer patients. As eminent Research Fellow of The Royal Society Dr Rupert Sheldrake reminds us, science should start from experience. Historically, successful treatments for cancer have always been around and we have recorded information about these throughout the 20th century, so we could reasonably expect the scientific and medical establishments to work with this information and determine the common denominators of the disease.

Dr Waltraut Fryda

Many years ago, I remember seeing a television programme which showed that cancer in rats completely disappeared when they were treated with something like adrenaline. I do not know why this particularly stuck in my mind, other than it seemed a revolutionary piece of research at the time. This memory was to be revived when I met Dr Fryda who had been practising her cancer treatment for over 40 years. Now retired, in the past she worked alone using local medical laboratories to carry out the necessary tests for her patients and did not have the time or resources to fund trials and produce statistics that the establishment might require. However, with her treatment she has healed very many patients with cancer. Over the years she has delivered papers and lectures on her hypothesis at many of the world's leading medical establishments, including the International Congress for Diseases of Civilization in Bregenz and The Viennese Medical Association. In addition, her publications, including research papers, are to be found in a variety of medical journals. Her method of treating cancer is not a magic bullet. It requires understanding, skill and technique. In this chapter I try to give a very simplified outline of Dr Fryda's hypothesis, which she has written about in her books *Adrenalinmangel als Ursache der Krebsentstehung*, and *Diagnose: Krebs* (available in English as *Diagnosis: Cancer*). [1]

Understanding the hypothesis

During my stay in Germany with Dr Fryda, I began to understand the way she worked with cancer. She briefly outlined her hypothesis to me, saying that in essence human beings are all similar and at the same time very individual, something which she acknowledges when treating her patients. (I found this very encouraging, it enabled me to draw a parallel with my own work and the fine-tuning to the individual). She revealed to me that cancer is a systemic disease, arriving as a result of ongoing stress factors. 'Stress' is a term bandied about a lot these days, and seems to cover a multitude of things, but in general terms we talk of being 'stressed' in relation to work and everyday pressures, which can also be emotional.

Stress factors in cancer

In the 21st century we are well overdue in expanding our under-standing of 'stress' in terms of its application to physical and mental health and – in this particular case – to cancer, as the list of stress factors can be very long, subtle and not necessarily as simple as 'over worked' or 'emotionally pressured'. 'One man's food is another man's poison,' is an old saying that has a lot of truth in it; it is an indicator of our individuality, telling us that what is good for one is not necessarily so for another. We all know that given a stressful situation, how we react and deal with it will vary from person to person. If we succumb to one type of stress it doesn't mean that we therefore succumb to all other similar stresses in the same way. Indeed, given a similar stress we may respond in a very robust 'water off a duck's back' kind of way. But what of the *hidden* stress factors around us, those that silently and anonymously impinge on our bodies; the hidden environmental, chemical and electromag-netic toxins which are also threatening the delicate balance of our health? Our endocrine system tempers and balances the hormones in our bodies; it is a delicate system which can be affected by numerous stress factors and adrenaline, the stress hormone, is there to help deal with these.

Adrenaline

The adrenal glands, which are about the size of two peas, sit at the top of the kidneys and are part of the chromaffin system. Hormone levels are generally measured in terms of being too high or too low, but in the case of adrenaline Dr Fryda realized that the medical establishment was only interested in the problems associated with too much of it. It was here that she began looking and found that those with cancer usually had very little adrenaline, often not registering at all on the accepted scale of measuring. Now she was able to track the significance of the role of adrenaline in the development of cancer.

In cancer, it appears that the tumour is the end result, not the beginning of the disease, which has usually developed over many years as the system has gradually become unable to cope or resist in the normal healthy way. Adrenaline, or rather the lack of it, is the key in Dr Fryda's hypothesis. First, we need to understand how the tumour arrives and the role of adrenaline.

Healthy adrenal response

Adrenaline is required in many situations and, as a stress hormone, it is the one which acts in the 'flight or fight' response, expanding the necessary blood vessels as it rushes to the part of the body urgently needing help, at the same time restricting blood vessels elsewhere in order to conserve energy where it is not needed.

When our body is invaded with bacteria or viruses and infections which make us feel ill, adrenaline rallies the body to create an inflammatory response. This is when we get a fever, run a high temperature and feel lousy, taking to our bed until the invader has been dealt with by the healthy immune system, and the fever has subsided.

A vital action of adrenaline is to interact with insulin in the cells. First, insulin comes from the blood to supply sugar (glycogen) to the cells. This 'energy' – the glycogen in the cells – is required for muscular activity; however, for the muscles to receive this energy, the glycogen must be released from the cells and the only way this can happen is with adrenaline. This is the healthy state, causing the body to produce right-turning (dextrorotatory) lactic acid, which is beneficial to the system and helps to balance the appropriate amount of adrenaline production.

Impaired adrenals

However, if we look at this from the point of view of an impaired adrenal response, it becomes very different. Let us now assume that the body has been slowly acquiring stress levels that have put a strain on the adrenals to the degree that they are unable to produce much adrenaline.

The first difference to notice is that the glycogen in the cells – which has been put there with insulin – can no longer be efficiently released as energy, because the level of adrenaline is low. This is unfortunate as adrenaline is the main hormone able to perform the task of releasing glycogen from the cells. Insulin carries on regardless, pushing more and more glycogen into the cells as that is its job. The cells are now overloaded with glycogen and no release is available due to the lack of adrenaline, and so the body begins to overproduce substitute hormones. In the case of the 'flight or fight' response, the missing adrenaline is substituted by the hormone noradrenaline, which is not made exclusively in the adrenals.

Here there are problems, as noradrenaline is unable to release glycogen from the cells and also responds to the 'flight or fight' by restricting *all* the blood vessels, unlike the more discriminating adrenaline which only restricts the unnecessary areas. This general constriction induces an overall lack of oxygen to the cells so that not only are the cells overloaded with glycogen, but they now are also deprived of oxygen.

As far as getting ill and developing a fever in order to deal with visiting infections is concerned, there is little healthy resistance available as the adrenals are not capable of producing enough resistance to induce a fever. Consequently, the likelihood of having a temperature to kill the infection and clear the system has become very slight.

The cells have now become weakened in their unhealthy state and, because of the effect of the insulin, the cells become porous, leaving them susceptible to viruses and bacteria. In order to deal with the glycogen overload the engorged cells are now forced to try to deal with the situation by resorting to a primitive form of fermentation and instead of producing the healthy right-turning lactic acid, they now produce the opposite, left-turning (laevorota-tory) lactic acid which is toxic to the system.

The beginning of the tumour

This toxic overload sets the perfect scene for instigating the division of cells, creating the cancer cells which are to form the tumour. More and more glycogen is used to fuel the tumour growth and for a time the patient has a levelling off in the progress of the disease as the glycogen has an outlet into the tumour. Later, with metastases appearing elsewhere, this leads to a hypoglycaemic condition as gradually the sugar resources are taken from wherever possible in the body, to fuel the tumour which has now created its own universe.

Reversing the process

This being the scenario, the route to health would logically be to reverse this process and this was my whole reason for spending seven weeks with Dr Fryda, in order to begin what would be at least a two to three year process. Goethe's statement, 'If you want to understand what something is, you must look and see where it came from,' is simple and logical. It is nothing sensational or out on a limb, just common sense. It also makes sense that, as the cancer has been a long-standing problem, the process of reversing the cancer and returning the body to a state of good health may also take time.

Whatever has been a stress or an irritation must be removed, and then orthodox medicine can be used to bring the system back to normal. Our levels of adrenaline fluctuate throughout the day according to the sophisticated fine-tuning of our bodies: conse-quently the regeneration injections are extremely subtle and given to help the body to regenerate its own adrenaline. This is the total opposite to dependency on harsh drugs to replace whatever is deficient. The use of such harsh drugs can easily destroy the body's own ability to ever again produce the very thing that it is lacking.

(Giving adrenaline injections to a patient is not possible because they can be extremely dangerous if administered inappropriately. Moreover, such injections have nothing to do with what is written about in this book.)

The regeneration is also for the immune system as well as the adrenals, and it is worth noting that, like the hormone melatonin, adrenaline levels drop off with age. These injections used in Germany are not available here in the UK. On my returning home, my UK doctor acknowledged that the injections were approved in the European Union, but not on the list in the UK. This being the case, it was up to me to supply and inject myself. In addition, a supplement of right-turning lactic acid was instrumental in the body regaining its proper body tissue and pH balance, as cancer patients have an acidic system which is part of the problem.

Naturally, foods with a high glycaemic index are not allowed. The injections continue for about a year, depending on the individual, and the diet and lactic acid for two years. After this the body has hopefully resumed normality and then it is most important to keep to a healthy diet for the rest of your life.

Life changes

In addition to diet, the numerous stress factors, whether physical, emotional, environmental or any other, have to be dealt with, and so this is the time for making life changes. Meditation on a regular basis is a great help in addressing both physical and mental problems and has been found to lower stress levels. The additional stress of long-standing chronic diseases such as allergies, low-grade infections and other aggravations need to be dealt with and cleared: yet another de-stress action, important in regaining full health.

A quick fix

A big problem nowadays is that whenever we get ill, our first response is to suppress the symptoms. Whether it is a cold, influenza or other minor upsets, we reach for the over-the-counter, quick-fix remedies, or go to the GP for yet another course of antibiotics, rather than allowing the illness to run its course. It is worth avoiding:

1 The use of over-the-counter remedies produced by the pharmaceutical giants which *suppress* the symptoms of an illness without rectifying the cause.
2 The liberal use of antibiotics and anti-inflammatories – the two most used (or abused) tools in the GP's armoury.
3 The highly effective publicity from the pharmaceutical companies through numerous television adverts to try and ensure that we buy their products for colds, headaches, indigestion and many other complaints.

Suppressing an illness by taking quick-fix remedies, or a constant stream of antibiotics which then enable you to carry on life as if you were well, does not allow the body to engage in a fever which would make it necessary to go to bed and let the immune system rise and fight, thereby strengthening itself. To suppress the illness might get you back to work quicker, but it does not serve your health in the long term.

Undermining the body's defences

As the facts about how cancer manifests in the body were revealed to me, it all made sense and removed my former assumption that we do not understand much about this disease. Clearly this is not the case. The whole idea of cancer so often developing over several years, as the system is put under the modern-day stresses and strains that are now considerably more abundant for both young and old than ever before, appears quite logical. During that time the body tries to combat the depletion in the normal way, until finally it is pushed over the critical margin and cancer or other diseases can no longer be eliminated from the system.

We all have cancer cells present in our bodies; it is a natural part of our existence in the same way as black and white, night and day, and good and bad. Cancer cells are present even at birth, so they are not strangers to our systems. Normally the complex, wonderful human constitution is able to deal with unwanted foreign cells through its immune system. But when cancer presents itself to an exhausted organism, not only are the adrenals depleted, but so are other aspects including the immune system.

Unravelling the disease

It would seem logical in the unravelling of cancer – i.e. reversing the process in order to bring the body back to good health – that the various aspects of depletion should be addressed together. Somehow, the magic bullet, although a wonderful idea, seems to miss the mark right now. Everyone is different and although there are general rules to be followed, each individual will have peculiarities that need addressing.

Finding depletions

Once I had arrived with Dr Fryda, extensive tests were taken and these had significant results. Along with the adrenaline, my thyroid level was found to be very low, common in women with breast cancer and often brushed aside in the UK as unimportant. In addition my selenium was down, one of the body's best defences against cancer. Dr Fryda prescribed a supplement of selenium, being careful to monitor the rise in subsequent tests until it reached a satisfactory level whereupon she gradually withdrew the supplement, believing that an overdose is dangerous and could be toxic to the liver. These and other aspects of the body chemistry were carefully addressed in my treatment and brought back into balance, to be further monitored in the following two years.

Why my body was so lacking in certain essentials seemed significant, not only in my treatment, but also with regard to the fact that I was eating in what I believed to be a healthy way. Once faced with the new diet and my eagerness to discover a better approach, I realized that I could make improvements; however, the environmental factor was one I had not seriously considered. It is a huge subject but appears to be very significant within the overall picture as our natural resources are now so very depleted. Even in the 1930s there was dismay at the erosion of minerals in our soil, a situation that has obviously worsened since. In addition, the high levels of pollution now surrounding us, combined with other stresses and strains, leave the body lacking in many of its daily requirements. We would hope that most of these necessities are met by having an organic diet, but it seems that it is not quite so simple. As I found later, even within the world of organic food there are variations in the levels of nutrition.

Turning the tide

During my seven weeks in Germany, through Dr Fryda's watchful eye and deep experience, a course was steered to begin the process of reversing the cancer. Five days a week I had injections to regenerate my system and I strictly adhered to the diet.

By the time I had reached the end of week five of the seven weeks, the process was expected to show the first signs of reversing the illness. With the additional help of lactic acid to enable the body to regain its natural pH balance, this is the point at which the blood/tissue levels return to a normal status and when a patient can feel a little out of sorts for a day or so. I can only say that it went by almost unnoticed, other patients finding much the same. Many people have asked me if the treatment has any nasty side effects, and there are none.

The golden mean

By the time my last tests were taken, near the end of the seven weeks, my cancer markers had made a quite dramatic drop into the range of 'normal'. I brought the prescribed injections back to the UK and continued administering one daily, five days a week, for the following three months. After three months, the injections were reduced to three a week, and by six months they became one a week – continuing until a year after the start of the treatment. After that, I was given the option of taking Iscador, a medicine made from the mistletoe plant, used frequently for breast cancer in Europe and now increasingly in the UK. However, it was not deemed necessary and consequently my regime was left to general maintenance of diet and any supplements that might be needed for a further twelve months. The diet became my great support and reading the small print on any food product became vital.

The adrenals took a while to respond – apparently this is not unusual. At fourteen months, my adrenaline had regenerated to a healthy level and I became aware of better energy. In order to maintain the 'golden mean' it became essential to have good sleep and regular exercise, to keep a general awareness of the body's needs, and to include regular meditation as it is more than purely the physical which needs to be taken care of. The crazy pace of living in a city, particularly London, demands that you regularly extract yourself from the merry-go-round and get back into your own skin. There is little doubt that those who are able to maintain the balance between both their inner and outer needs have a far greater chance of achieving good health, enjoying themselves and contributing positively in society.

Cancer acknowledged as a systemic disease

There are many other doctors and research scientists who regard cancer as a systemic disease which has its beginnings in stress, whether physical, viral, chemical or psychological, and they too recognize the need for the body to regenerate and reverse cancer. In 1998 the *American Journal of Natural Medicine* published a report by Robert A. Ronzio, PhD, CNS, FAIC, entitled 'Nutritional Support for Adrenal Function'. Ronzio quotes Hans Seyle – sometimes referred to as 'the Einstein of medicine' and creator of the term 'stress syndrome' – as saying that 'stress is life, and life is stress.' Ronzio goes on to say that it is the sustained day-to-day stress which alters the metabolism. Adapting to chronic stress, the pituitary gland responds, and so in turn do the adrenals, by producing elevated blood cortisol levels. By way of compensating, the hypothalamus and pituitary become less sensitive to the cortisol feedback inhibition. Insulin resistance increases. High cortisol and low DHEA will suppress the immune system. Eventually this leads to adrenal exhaustion. He says:

> Excessive fatigue, reduced ability to concentrate, alcohol intolerance, headache, menstrual irregularities, low blood pressure, reactive hypoglycemia and carbohydrate sensitivity may follow... In addition, acute stress amplifies liver detoxification enzymes and oxidative stress. This maladaption stage promotes chronic inflammation, tissue damage, and degenerative diseases ... The benefits of neonatal bovine adrenal preparations are noted as a regeneration, plus thymic extracts ... By analogy with thymic extracts, preparations of the hypothalamus/pituitary complex normalize endocrine functions. Indeed hypothalamic extracts induced the production of thymic peptides in aged mice [2]

Ronzio suggests nutritional support of B complex minerals as well as antioxidants including vitamin C, and gives information on the decline with age in adrenal vitamin C levels. He recommends that healthy unstressed young men require at least 200mg of vitamin C daily in order to saturate immune cells – far in excess of the current recommended daily allowance (RDA). It is interesting to note that beta-carotene is the major carotenoid found in the adrenals, and he suggests that natural sources of food are better than a supplement. (I found this information explained the large amount of carrot juicing recommended in many therapies.)

In an interview with Tashi Grady Powers in April 2004, Walter Last said:

> Chronic stress is the key. It leads to weakness and later exhaustion of the adrenal glands and deterioration of the hormonal and immune system, and is expressed as disease and early aging. We live in a minefield of chronic stress generators, such as eating cooked food, drinking

chlorinated or fluoridated water, breathing polluted air, using fluorescent lighting, wearing synthetic clothing, having mercury in teeth, worrying or being apprehensive of something, and on and on it goes.

We are rarely stress free, even while sleeping we may be still under the influence of drugs, and exposed to harmful magnetic fields. Chronic stress has explosively increased over the last century. We need to discover the important stress generators that affect us personally and try to minimize them, while at the same time maximizing stress protectors, such as fresh raw food, enjoyable activities, especially in fresh air and natural surroundings, meditation, and positive social interactions.

I believe that the human body has an almost unlimited capacity to regenerate and, therefore, has no fixed age limit. With this, I believe that it is natural for us to live free of disease, and full of mental and physical abilities until our soul decides to depart. Presently diseases and aging are the norm because we do not live in harmony with our biological, social and spiritual nature. We can more or less reverse our present health deterioration by improving harmony on all of these levels as part of our spiritual journey. Our personal health, emotional and mental problems can show us what we need to do in order to become more harmonious and, with this, more healthy and whole. I direct my energies towards finding and teaching methods that everyone can use in this endeavor, and move towards increasing levels of harmony on all levels of our existence. [3]

A route to conquering cancer

As long ago as 1950, the vision of where we should be aiming in the search for health and the cure of cancer was quite clear. Dr Max Gerson, MD (1881–1959) whose work still continues in South

America and many other parts of the world, successfully treated thousands of cancer patients through diet and nutrition. He was well aware of the direction we need to take in the 21st century, saying,

> I am convinced that the problem of chronic diseases is not one of biochemistry, chemistry or the symptoms we observe in and on the body. Rather, it is produced by deeper-lying forces which cause 'deficiency of energies' ... The real acting forces behind the visible chemical changes are physical energies, expressed by Einstein as the electromagnetic field.

Reversing cancer

Roger Coghill, who runs Coghill Research Laboratories in Wales, is one of the UK's leading scientists researching into the hazards of electromagnetic fields (EMFs). In a paper titled 'Reassessing Koch's reagents and the potency of melatonin', published in the March 2004 edition of the *Institute for Complementary Medicine Journal*, Coghill examined the work that William Koch, the Professor of Physiology at what is now Wayne State University, USA, had carried out in the 1920s:

> Koch, like Nobel Prize winners Otto Warburg and Albert Szent-Gyorgyi decades after him, believed that cancer was a result of faulty mechanism and that it might be possible to return the malignant cells to normality. He was evidently right. In the decade between 1920 and 1929, when his reagents became the principal cancer treatment in Detroit, his home city, cancer mortality there fell by 23%, whilst in every other major US city it was rising by as much as 32% during that decade. So how did Koch single-handedly manage to achieve what no subsequent multi-million cancer programmes have ever done?

In his report, Coghill identifies the same contributory factors as the others already mentioned in this chapter. The cancer cell has a great need for glucose and has poor oxygen uptake. In the further stages of the breakdown, viral or chemical interference to the cell causes it to rely on glycosis alone for survival. The cell craves glucose, goes on a hunt to the epithelial tissue in order to proliferate, growing into a tumour with its own blood supply and impenetrable to the T-cells (killer cells): this is how it develops. He goes on to talk of scientist Dr Karl Folkers' discovery of the role of ubiquinone in the 1950s, which led to what is now known as CoQ10 (which is readily available as a supplement). Koch took this further by harnessing other, superior aspects of quinones which dehydrogenated the carcinogens more efficiently, and so caused a chain reaction through the body, dislodging these carcinogens which then became neutralized. Most importantly, Koch's reagents had not killed the cell (as in our current methods of cut, poison and burn), but had reversed or unravelled the procedure back to normality. Many of his patients were in good health thirty years later and yet had required only one intramuscular or sublingual dose to achieve this. Hundreds of long-term successes were recorded, along with spectacularly successful animal trials. However, the pharmaceutical industry was not interested as Koch's process was not patentable.

Coghill goes on to state how simply a faulty metabolism of glucose in which the cell becomes starved of oxygen can cause glycosis even without carcinogens. By simply depriving normal cells of oxygen, they produced cells indistinguishable from cancer cells. He also points out that the human breast is poorly vascularized (it does not have a great blood supply), so even a slight bruise can induce this situation. On this basis it is not difficult to see how smoking can inhibit oxygenation, a stress which could then lead to lung cancer.

In the light of this information and considering the delicacy of the human breast, it goes against all logic to squash the breast in a mammogram machine, and indicates that women must take care to protect their breasts in some of the more aggressive body-contact sports that are now popular.

Taking once again the approach of Koch, Coghill, with his understanding of electro-pathways in cells, is already producing promising results whilst at the same time a privately financed team in Budapest including Jakab and Schoenfeld is also carrying out trials. [4]

Conclusion

Born of a need to understand my own illness, this consensus of research brought me to acknowledge that the health of the adrenal, hormonal (endocrine) and immune systems is a golden key to unravelling this disease. The removal of stress and detrimental environmental factors and the balancing of our lives, both physically and emotionally, play a vital part in becoming healthy and whole. So rather than searching for a magic bullet – a phrase ringing with the violence of a gunshot – wouldn't it be so much better to use the golden key which can unlock this disease, allowing a reversal of the cancer, rather than confronting the body with a 'shot' in order to destroy it, and at the same time endanger the healthy parts of the body?

13 Our Environment

The great majority of chemicals released into our environment, including those used in our food, toiletries, cosmetics and household products are not tested or regulated for carcinogenicity. A report in the *Ecologist* in October 2000 tells us that, up until World War II, investigators searched for carcinogens not only in the atmosphere, but in food, alcohol and occupational materials. The concern now is that the expanding dominance of industry and business over our society has, over the last 50 years, increasingly pushed the responsibility for environmental illnesses, including cancer, onto the individual suffering from the disease. If the cause of cancer is not genetic, then it is seen to be the fault of the individual.[1] However, most of us are aware that, whatever these financially driven businesses and industries provide for us, we are neither consulted nor given a choice in the matter of testing for carcinogens in their products. It is deeply worrying that these problems have been growing unchecked for many decades.

Soil deficiency

It was as far back as the 1930s that the US government expressed concerns about the effect the depletion of vital nutrients in the soil was having on US citizens:

> Do you know that most of us today are suffering from

certain dangerous diet deficiencies which cannot be remedied until depleted soils from which our food comes are brought into proper balance? Our physical well-being is more directly dependent upon minerals we take into our systems than upon calories or vitamins, or upon precise proportions of starch, protein or carbohydrates we consume.

It is bad news to learn from our leading authorities that 99 per cent of the American people are deficient in these minerals, and that a marked deficiency in any one of the more important minerals actually results in disease.

Any upset of the balance, any considerable lack of one or other element, however microscopic the body requirements may be, and we sicken, suffer and shorten our lives.

Whether you eat a balanced diet or not you are probably malnourished. This fact has been known for over 60 years but we have not been warned or given information to help us correct the deficiencies. With improper nutrients and minerals we have weakened immune systems.[2]

Statements such as this are examples of governments recognizing problems raised by scientific research, and noting that action needs to be taken. But the action never materializes. This worldwide problem is ongoing and showing no signs of being rectified, as further damage to our health and the environment continues. Here, in the UK, Dr B Durrant-Peatfield reminds us that in the US in 1997 the National Academy of Sciences (NAS) confirmed that most Americans are magnesium deficient.[3] I have quoted these reports from the USA because information on the present state of the soil in the UK seems very difficult to find. During my research in 2004, the most up-to-date information I could find was a graph of 1995 from the Department of the Environment, showing the levels of organic topsoil up to 1995 when the topsoil was down to about 7 per cent and gradually reducing. Unlike in the USA, this kind of information is not easily available in the UK. The Department for the Environment directed me to Cranfield University which specializes in soil analysis, where I was told that funding for soil research was stopped some years ago as there was very little interest shown in the UK. However, there has been an uptake of interest in the last few years which has revealed that not only do parts of north and west Norfolk now have an organic topsoil of less than 1 per cent, but generally there is widespread pollution. Many UK farmers are adding to the problem by putting far too much sewage on crops.

As for soil research, it is outsourced by the UK Government, but just how the information is collated and dealt with poses questions as to how well we are being served. Richard Young of the Soil Association tells us that 'we are only left with industry-funded research, or no research at all. There are very few academics who aren't beholden in some way to industry.' He goes on to say, 'These bodies are not independent at all. From the universities, to the food producers, to the product regulators, the pharmaceutical companies have their fingers in every pie.'

Chemicals, genetics and cancer

Young points out that since 1982 cattle have had, by law, to be treated for warble fly with Phosmet, an organophosphate pesticide. What is perhaps not so widely known is that Phosmet was developed by Nazi chemists in World War II as a chemical weapon nerve agent. Later, Phosmet was marketed as an agricultural pesticide by ICI, and afterwards by its renamed pharmaceutical subdivision, Zeneca. Many studies have shown that organophosphates bring health risks and that DNA can be damaged by chemicals: damaged DNA is directly connected to cancer. The use of such harmful chemicals in the natural environment poses many questions. Considering that about 93 per cent of breast cancer is *not* genetic, why is there such a huge proportion of research dealing with genetic cancer – therefore not serving the vast majority of women? For example, what research is going into the problem of carcinogens in the soil – a problem compounded by the use of pesticides, many of which are well recognized as playing a part in cancer and other illnesses? Professor Andrew Watterson, addressing the public meeting in Boston in 2001 (*see* page 135) said:

> Research programmes on breast cancer are all focussed on genetics. It seems that if you have a genetic susceptibility to cancer, the researchers can deal with it. In the NHS cancer plan there is a reference to smoking and a reference to diet. That's all. But we have 170 pesticides all of which are carcinogenic in animals and suspected to be carcinogenic in humans.[4]

Sir Richard Body, who chaired the 1987 House of Commons Agriculture Committee hearing which led to the Body Report – *The Effects of Pesticides on Human Health* – was also one of the speakers at the Boston conference. He recalled being in Brussels, browsing through the Yellow Pages, coming across chemical companies and recognizing 12 international names. He noticed the addresses were close to the headquarters of the European Commission. They were not manufacturing, marketing or selling there; these were the lobbying posts of these companies, employing skilful men and women who get to know the officials in the EU in order to influence them regarding the regulations. He sees this as one of the reasons why, on this side of the Atlantic, we have made so little progress in highlighting the dangers of pesticides.

Genetically modified organisms (GMOs)

The UK Environment Agency is described thus: 'The leading public body for protecting and improving the environment in England and Wales, the Environment Agency's responsibilities are wide-ranging. It has powers to regulate air pollution, land quality and waste management, water quality and use, builds flood defences and provides flood warnings.' It is listed as a product and service government body. The names of these government organizations appear to change quite frequently, causing confusion not only to the public, but also to those who work in them. Sixteen years ago, long before the Environment Agency came into existence, a report from what was then called the Ministry for Agriculture, Fisheries and Food (MAFF) gave vital information to the UK government on the subject of genetically modified organisms (GMOs), which appears to have been ignored. 'New Scientific Findings Confirming Fears Over Health Hazards of GMOs' was a MAFF letter to their Joint Food, Safety and Standards Group in 1998. The letter highlighted the transfer of antibiotic marker genes to environmental organisms and, amongst others, the transfer of transgenic DNA into mammalian cells. If, as the present UK government proposes, the GMO issue is allowed to go ahead, then this decision will be another instance of research which clearly shows dangers yet again being ignored, and ultimately wasted. Inevitably this will add to the already complex problem of cancer and its causes from the environment.

The journalist Rebecca Fowler pointed out that in Canada the disaster of GM crops has driven farming communities to revert to using highly toxic chemicals on their crops in order to hold back 'superweeds' caused by wild plants which have been infected with herbicide-resistant genes from GM crops. As she points out, this problem passes down the food chain to us and at the same time the chemical-pharmaceutical industry makes a great deal of money.[5]

The body and chemical disrupters

In the UK, Dr Rosy Daniel is one of several who have voiced their fears. She believes that a great deal of cancer is caused through our food chain, a consequence of chemical and biological changes in today's highly processed food.[6]

Professor Andrew Watterson, who found that trying to access the Department of Health's website for information on breast cancer and the environment was a lost cause, tells us that:

The concerns about endocrine disrupting chemicals have changed the ground rules internationally on how we control these chemicals. The assumptions the regulators have made up to now have been: we can set the standards, we can use the chemicals safely, there won't be interactions, we know what the levels are, and even when we don't we can be sure that the levels won't hurt us, pollution problems can be solved because even if chemicals get to the Arctic they will be diluted – but the scientific evidence makes a nonsense of that – and that human activity is local, not global. But with the endocrine disrupting chemicals the accepted form of toxicology has gone out of the window. The precautionary principle should be the starting point.[7]

Oestrogen

With chemical pollutants, the situation can arise where the body's hormone receptors do not differentiate its own biological oestrogens from man-made oestrogens. Information that has recently been brought to our attention suggests that this situation is compounded by the highly dangerous overuse of antibiotics fed to cattle grazing on land which is full of pesticides. Consider this, plus the growth-boosting hormones to be found in meat and dairy products, and it should be enough to convert us all to eating only organic food.

Chemicals and the effects on women's bodies

Cynthia Wilson points out that old people and children are usually regarded as the vulnerable in society, but believes this may be missing the point when it comes to chemicals because the most vulnerable may be women. Natural oestrogens are greater in women's bodies than men's with their biosynthetic pathways being more vulnerable, this vulnerability further increasing when women take birth control pills. Releasing toxins from the system is primarily done by the P450 enzyme system which is part of a more complex metabolic system that is highly vulnerable to chemicals. Cynthia Wilson points out that chemical oestrogens can impact on these systems, inhibiting or completely inactivating them, and that illnesses related to this breakdown are first and foremost a women's issue. [8]

This view is reinforced by Sarah Sexton who reveals that egg and sperm cells, an embryo at 0–8 weeks, a foetus at 9–40 weeks, a young child and also reproductive and sexual organs, can all be damaged by industrial chemicals, depending on the timing.[9]

Adding weight to these findings, Dr Philippa Darbre tells us

> Epidemiology shows that 90 per cent of breast cancers are environmental in origin and linked to a Western lifestyle, but the specific environmental causes have never been identified. Around five to ten per cent of breast cancer arises from genetic susceptibility, but the question remains as to susceptibility to what? The main identified risk factors relate to lifetime exposure to the female hormone oestrogen, through variations in puberty, menopause, childbirth and personal choices such as use of the contraceptive pill or hormone replacement therapy. Diet, smoking and excessive alcohol consumption can also have an effect. However it is estimated that there remain still seventy per cent of breast cancers unaccounted for by these known risk factors … DNA can also be damaged by radiation and by chemicals, and here may lie the reason for the enormity of the rise in breast cancer over recent years. The question is which. Radiation or chemicals? … a variety of agrochemicals and industrial pollutants can accumulate in body tissues and because many are fat-soluble they can accumulate over a lifetime very effectively in breast fat. … some of these chemicals, such as DDT and PCBs can also mimic the action of oestrogen, and oestrogen is well known to play a role in development of breast cancer. … breast

cancer can arise many years before lumps become visible,
making it impossible to know the real measurement of
chemicals when the initiating events actually happened.
… With PCBs for example, there are 209 different forms.
It is almost impossible to know which of the thousands of
chemicals are really important to measure. Therefore we
are left with inconclusive data where some studies
conclude more DDT or PCB in women with breast
cancer and some do not. There is a real danger of not
being able to give these chemicals a fair trial. And, of
course, these chemicals remain innocent until proven
guilty. That is the dilemma of the scientist.[10]

When we are informed as succinctly as this, we have to acknowledge
those scientists who strive for the good and implore our governments and politicians to support research which, above all, is not
related to industry and money. How sensitive the human system and
how instinctive and wise these research scientists have to be! It
surely highlights the enormous need to respect and understand
both the body and the environment we live in, before making environmental changes that could cause terrible harm. It is tragic that
many of these changes, or 'developments', have been going on
unmonitored for far too long and at the cost of human life.

Transparency of research

The USA appears to be more open and honest and more ready
than many countries to admit to a lack of research on certain major
cancer issues. The Finns are amongst others who are also more
open and honest, and their record for health and safety is the worst,
as they reckon around 40 per cent of the workforce is affected by
chemicals, some of which are carcinogens. The Finns keep the best
records and have the toughest standards, showing a transparency
which leaves the UK way behind. It would be helpful if the UK
authorities showed a similar willingness for transparency where
both cancer and electromagnetic pollution are concerned.

Electromagnetic pollution

We are now living in an electromagnetic smog. What effect does this have on our health? Thomas Saunders tells us that exposure to low-frequency electromagnetic fields can reduce melatonin level secretions by as much as 50 per cent.

> Radio and microwave frequencies can pass through buildings and all other obstacles including our flesh, blood, organs and brain ... the Environmental Health Criteria 137 published by the World Health Organization (WHO) in 1993 warned that radio frequency radiation for transmitters can have a similar hazardous effect as living under power lines. The report says 'There is increasing concern about the possibility that radio frequency exposure may play a role in the causation or promotion of cancer, specifically of the blood forming organs or in the central nervous system. Similar uncertainties surround possible effects on reproduction, such as increased rates of spontaneous abortion and congenital malformations. At frequencies below a few hundred kilohertz, the electrical stimulation of excitable membranes of nerves and muscle cells is a well established phenomenon.'[11]

Further investigations in the USA into these problems have also proved positive. Again, we find that the amount of research in the UK by the government body, the National Radiological Protection Board (NRPB), is lower than in other countries, and yet it is common knowledge that clusters of cancers have occurred in some areas where radio frequency transmitters are to be found. Despite the evidence, in the UK cellular phone companies can erect masts and antennae more or less anywhere they choose. Thomas Saunders also tells us that the British Ministry of Defence research on radio frequencies and microwaves is being kept secret and that most other major countries take the risks of electromagnetic problems much more seriously. The levels of radiation allowed by other governments are often much lower than those in the UK.

Oestrogens and EMF pollutants

Just as most people can understand that it may be unwise to build your home next to an overhead electricity pylon, very few people are aware that it is often the extremely small electromagnetic fields (EMFs) that can be the most harmful. Mobile phones have raised this awareness, but those who have researched deeply into the problem know that there are serious risks with mobile phones that the National Radiological Protection Board prefers not to acknowledge. The fact is that small amounts of EMFs can mimic the body's own electromagnetic field and consequently cause chaos by fooling the body into believing that they 'naturally' belong there. It is a similar story to that of the artificial and chemically induced oestrogens. In April 1992 the *Electronics World and Wireless World* reported that:

> ... considerable evidence indicates that low-frequency electronic and magnetic fields coinciding with natural ion magnetic resonances can have a biological effect on the pineal gland. Human blood contains ions that have a range of resonance with the Earth's geomagnetic field and an alternating field ranging between 1Hz and 500Hz. If an electrical or magnetic field is applied near this resonance frequency it can impact upon the lymphocyte cells which, in turn, will affect the immune system response and may well explain many cases of lymphatic leukaemia and other diseases.

As so many men and women of all ages, even young children, carry mobile phones on standby most of the time, research is warning us of the hazards and advises switching on only when necessary.

Thomas Saunders points out that a report from a Forestry

Commission study as long ago as 1993 revealed that trees that had healthy root systems were found to be dying from the top down: all of them within a few kilometres of high-powered multi-use radio and microwave masts.[12]

Possible danger from an underwired bra

He goes on to mention that Ann Silk, ophthalmologist and Fellow of the Royal Society of Medicine was one of the investigators who, in her research into the possible causes of breast cancer, suggested that the wires in the underwiring of women's bras could act as re-radiating antennae.

Although they are relatively new, it is now possible to buy an underwired bra that uses plastic instead of wiring, counteracting a possible problem.

Toxic dangers in the effects of perfume both externally and internally

It seems extraordinary that there is no agency in existence to regulate the fragrance industry. These products penetrate the skin and can affect the organs in the body. They also saturate the bloodstream, and the body then has to work to clear the toxins. In other words this is another stress factor for the body. There appears to be evidence that they can cause discolouring of internal organs. Also, the so-called 'natural' products and perfumes can be suspect, not only because of their content, but, rather like the food issue, because of the way in which they are processed. Research has shown a connection between the early use of antiperspirants and deodorants and underarm shaving to an earlier age of breast cancer diagnosis. A graph of deodorant and antiperspirant sales mirrored the rise in breast cancer and gave 90 per cent as the figure for people in the US using these toiletries.[13]

This alone has to be valid confirmation of Dr Philippa Darbre's research in the UK, condemning deodorants as dangerous, especially as she informs us that there is now a disproportionately large incidence of breast cancer in the upper, outer quadrant of the breast, where these products are applied.

Parabens in cosmetics and toiletries

Since parabens have now been shown to be able to mimic the action of the female hormone oestrogen and to get into the human breast, this poses some important questions over their use in consumer products, especially cosmetic products applied around the breast area. Some of their common names are: methylparaben, propylparaben, ethylparaben and butylparaben. Deodorants, perfumes and toiletries have had a question mark hanging over them for some time, but thanks to the work of Dr Darbre we are now beginning to get an informed picture. This raises the question of why parabens are also added as preservatives to thousands of foods, cosmetics, pharmaceuticals and some anti-cancer drugs. It is only recently that this very important issue has come to light: no doubt those with a financial interest in these industries will be quick to assure us that there is not a problem.

Dr Darbre won't use any of these products, organic or otherwise, and recommends washing twice a day, telling us that:

> Women apply increasing chemical loads under their arms and around their breasts including body lotions, body creams, breast firming creams, breast enhancing creams, shaving creams, tanning creams, sun-care creams etc.

Quite an awesome list when you think about it. Dr Darbre points out that there is accumulating evidence of the toxicity of components of these cosmetics and, in the final analysis, it will be chemical overload versus individual susceptibility.

One woman, who no longer uses a deodorant, said that after a while she found her body had 'acclimatized' and the less she used a deodorant, the less she needed one. It may come as rather a tall order to some of us to totally abandon a deodorant or an antiperspirant, in which case I advise you to read 'Toxic Toiletries' in *What*

Doctors Don't Tell You.[14] The authors suggest that when choosing a personal care product, 'If you can't put it *in* your body, don't put it *on* your body.'

In the case of creams and lotions, it is not difficult to see how any of these products, when applied to the body, might have an effect internally. By regularly rubbing a small amount of natural progesterone cream into the skin, it is absorbed into the bloodstream and progesterone levels in the blood increase. It can be easy to ignore such a simple fact when it is beneficial to our health, but quite alarming when you consider how treacherous the regular use of cosmetics might be. At the very least, we should search out natural products and read the small print.

Sunscreens

The market for sunscreens is highly lucrative with an increasingly large number of products available, yet it seems very likely that the application of sunscreens prevents the body from synthesizing adequate amounts of vitamin D, as well as encouraging us to stay in the sun for dangerously long periods of time. Added to this, the contents of a sunscreen give rise to the question of safety, as many of them contain parabens and toxic chemicals commonly found in toiletries. Natural oils from plants have often been used by those living in hotter climates, but for many of us who only get a chance to sunbathe on our annual holiday, we automatically look for a sunscreen with the greatest protection.

UVB and UVA filters

There has been much confusion in recent years about UVB and UVA filters in these products and the sun protection (SP) factors. The problem seems to lie in most sun lotions not protecting in equal amounts against UVB and UVA, the UVA filter being less stable and disintegrating when applied to the skin. Research has shown that it is the UVA rays that penetrate most deeply and are around in considerable strength during the sunshine hours of the day, peaking at midday. UVB rays are strongest at midday also, but have a much more significant tail-off either side. Dr Mark Porter, the health and fitness correspondent for the *Evening Standard*, suggests buying the highest UVA protection, for example, an SPF 15 with a UVA of 4 stars or more. [15]

Sunscreens and cancer

Whilst sunscreens appear to be linked to the cancer problem, the good news is that the sun is highly beneficial to us and we need it. In Dr Richard Hobday's excellent book, *The Healing Sun – Sunlight and Health in the 21st Century*, he refers to this report by Drs Frank and Cedric Garland.

> Worldwide, the countries where chemical sunscreens have been recommended and adopted have experienced the greatest rise in malignant melanoma, with a contemporaneous rise in death rates. In the United States, Canada, Australia, and the Scandinavian countries, melanoma rates have risen steeply in recent decades with the greatest increase occurring after the introduction of sunscreens. Death rates in the US from melanoma doubled in women and tripled in men between the 1950s and the 1990s. The rise in melanoma has been unusually steep in Queensland, Australia where sunscreens were earliest and most strongly promoted by the medical community. Queensland now has the highest incidence rate of melanoma in the world. In contrast, the rise in melanoma rates was notably delayed elsewhere in Australia, where sunscreens were not promoted until more recently.[16]

Benefits of the sun

The vast majority of us joyfully welcome the uplifting warmth and brightness of a sunny day, but for a long time we have been warned of the dangers of the sun and that it can be the cause of cancer.

Research tells us this is not so, and it is pleasing to know that sunbathing with discrimination is positively beneficial to our health. To be in the sun purely for your health is an approach that seems to have been almost lost in our current way of life, but Hobday's book reveals how, in the past, the sun has been used as a restorative, regenerating form of healing, able to conquer many diseases when, as with all cures, it is used with integrity. A sunlight therapist was awarded the Nobel Prize for Medicine in 1903, at a time when the reversal of damage by tuberculosis and the speedy healing of wounds were achieved by sunlight. Scientists knew that the therapy worked, but could not explain it.

> There is little scientific or, for that matter, historical evidence to support public health campaigns which recommend avoidance of the sun. There is no proof that sunlight causes melanoma, or that sunscreens prevent it. People who work indoors are at a greater risk of developing the disease than those who work outdoors and melanoma tends to occur on parts of the body less frequently exposed to sunlight such as the trunk and the back of the legs … a lifetime spent out in the sun decreases the risk of developing the disease … Vitamin D deficiency is implicated in a number of cancers and other major diseases. The action of sunlight on the skin is the natural way of producing vitamin D. So it is entirely plausible that the number of people who die each year of cancer of the breast, colon and prostate together with those who die from coronary heart disease, stroke and broken hips could be reduced by the adoption of regular, moderate sunbathing.[17]

Dr Hobday suggests that by putting babies out in the sun and sunlight, we are protecting them in childhood against later disease such as prostate cancer, multiple sclerosis and coronary heart disease. As children, many of us may remember being given a daily spoonful of cod liver oil. This is recommended to both young and old as a good source of the vital vitamin D which the sun normally provides but is lacking for a substantial part of the year in countries in the northern hemisphere. The body needs the sun to synthesize vitamin D, whereas diseases such as breast and prostate cancer, rickets, TB and osteoporosis suggest low levels of vitamin D. Clearly, we can benefit from the healing rays of the sun and it is worth knowing that the tuberculosis patients undergoing helio-therapy in the early twentieth century, were not considered to be healed unless they had a light tan.[18]

How can we protect ourselves?

Food and drink

Awesome as the task may seem to find a 'safe' way to shop when presented with the vast choice in food that is now available, there are many ways in which you can reasonably help protect yourself. First, acquire the habit of carefully reading the labels and buying high quality organic food wherever possible. Avoid pre-packed foods, not only because of the plastics that wrap them – or you venture down the road of artificial oestrogens – but also because of chemicals and other additives, often sugars which, amongst other things, appear to contribute to the huge increase in adult-onset diabetes, thereby opening the door to possible cancer. It is far better to buy fresh, local and seasonal foods. Highly processed foods are unnecessary, and when confronted with what might appear to be a healthy-looking product it is advisable to check the contents carefully. Avoid hydrogenated fats, present in many cakes and bread products and choose non-hydrogenated, cold-pressed cooking oils. Drink bottled or filtered water. Some people recommend boiling filtered or tap water because potentially toxic chemicals, chlorine, fluoride and artificial oestrogens, which are all recognized as creating health problems, are to be found in most tap water. Fruit drinks are usually full of sugar, so opt for pure fruit juice or juices sweetened with other fruits rather than with added sweeteners. If children feel deprived of fizzy drinks, a good solution is to add some of the sweeter fruits – such as pineapple – to carbonated water while their taste buds adapt to less sugar. Take care with the alcohol you consume as many cheaper wines, particularly white wines, have high acidity levels. Some of the best wines I have tasted have been organic-biodynamic.

Home and work

Use environment-friendly cleaning materials for the home and keep fresh air circulating throughout as levels of pollution in the home have been found to be very high. Use herbs, flowers and natural oils rather than artificial air-fresheners as many of the latter contain toxins. Natural materials are healthier for the furnishing of the home and work environment and both places require a good amount of daylight streaming through, so it is preferable to have large, clear windows. Avoid tinted glass as this prevents us from receiving normal daylight which the body needs to keep a balance in the pituitary and endocrine system. Artificial lighting also causes stress to the body, so avoid fluorescent lights or, where possible, opt for full-spectrum daylight lighting. At home, uncluttered rooms decorated in colours which bring you peace and relaxation are essential. There is now much more information available on colour and how it affects us, so if you are choosing decorations for the home or office it is a good idea to look carefully into what will be most beneficial. If you have a garden, be cautious about the fertilizer and growth-promoting products that you might use: check the contents carefully to see that they are not toxic.

Power lines and mobile phones

Avoid living near overhead power lines or pylons and check that there are no mobile phone masts on nearby buildings when choosing the best place to live. If you are faced with the possibility of mobile phone or TETRA masts being erected near you, campaign to stop them – it can be done and has been done. Get a good attachable protector for your mobile phone and use the phone to the minimum.

Personal care

Opt for a bra that is not underwired, or find one that is made with newer materials which will not have the chance to interact with radiation from mobile phones and other electromagnetic fields. Use natural materials for your clothing and non-toxic make-up and toiletries. Take plenty of fresh air and exercise regularly, recognizing the fact that the sun *is* healthy and we need it!

A useful checklist

Samuel Epstein MD, Emeritus Professor of Environmental and Occupational Medicine, University of Illinois at Chicago School of Public Health, and Chairman of the Cancer Prevention Coalition, provides us with a helpful summary of the most essential factors to be aware of in protecting ourselves. In his endorsement of the proposal by the Women's Environmental Network (WEN) and the Ban Lindane Campaign to develop a strategy for the primary prevention of breast cancer, presented to the UK All Party Parliamentary Group Meeting on Breast Cancer, 15 January 2002 he said:

> There are a wide range of well-developed avoidable breast cancer risk factors, information of which has not yet been made available to the public. These risk factors fall into three major categories as follows:

> **Medical**
> - Oral contraceptives, with early and prolonged use
> - Oestrogen replacement therapy, with high doses and prolonged use
> - Premenopausal mammography, with early and repeated radiation exposure
> - Non-hormonal prescription drugs, such as antihypertensives

- Silicone gel breast implants, especially those wrapped in polyurethane foam

Industrial
- Diets high in animal fat contaminated with carcinogenic pesticides, industrial contaminants, and oestrogenic cattle feed additives
- Diets high in dairy products contaminated with carcinogenic industrial contaminants, and genetically engineered rBGH (BST) milk
- Domestic exposure to carcinogenic household products, or pollutants from nearby chemical plants or hazardous waste sites
- Exposure to a wide range of occupational carcinogens

Lifestyle
- Nulliparity [*not having a baby*]
- Alcohol, with early and excessive use
- Tobacco, with early and excessive use
- Inactivity and sedentary lifestyle
- Black or brown permanent or semi-permanent hair dyes, with early and prolonged use.

14 Alternatives to Mammography

The question that every woman would like the answer to is, 'what alternatives are there to mammograms?' As we shall see, there are other options, but ultrasound seems the most readily available. Yet in spite of many GPs being suspicious of the safety of mammograms for conventional breast cancer screening, I know of several women aged 50 and over who have asked their doctors for ultrasound as an alternative – believing it to be safer – but have had their requests refused.

In a conversation with the administration department of the NHS Breast Screening Programme in 2006, I was told that doctors still follow the guidelines set out in the 1988 Forrest Report, which assessed its findings purely on clinical examination (palpation) and mammography. Still adhering to this report, the normal procedure, as in the guidelines set out for doctors, appears to be that a woman *must* have a mammogram first. This might possibly explain why it is not unusual for doctors to be angry at these requests for alternative imaging – deeply upsetting for the woman – whilst some women, who have already had breast cancer, are sometimes bullied by doctors into having a mammogram, usually annually. This outdated report seems to take precedence over the implementation of safer alternative methods for conventional breast cancer screening.

Fortunately, in many areas of science and medicine there are people who strive to move forward and make improvements for the benefit of us all. Much of the information in this chapter is drawn from research done by specialist doctors and scientists who, working in the medical establishment, have run trials and provided their colleagues in the world of medicine with the results which are printed in recognized medical journals.

Ultrasound

In 2001, a team from Addenbrooke's Hospital in Cambridge, UK, published research that informed us of several advantages to be found with ultrasound when compared to mammography, and revealed how the newer ultrasound models were also capable of showing breast calcifications. The objective of their research was to compare ultrasonography with mammography in 149 women who had a moderate family history of breast cancer. The average age of the women was just over 42 years.

The results were quite clear. The mammograms showed normal in 148 out of the 149 women. The ultrasound showed ten focal solid lesions which were biopsied as a result. One woman was found to have a lymph node and two women to have lesions which had previously been biopsied and shown to be benign, and 46 women had cysts. The other 90 women were normal. The report concluded that screening with both ultrasound and mammography in those with an increased risk of breast cancer might be beneficial and suggested further study was needed to examine how acceptable, reproducible and cost-effective it might be. The authors of the report pointed out that this was a pilot study and that the group was small.[1]

I have come to understand that whilst scientists and doctors strive to bring this sort of invaluable research to the attention of the medical establishment, they have to pander to the niceties of professional etiquette and show due deference to the 'system', presumably in order to be heard. If you or I were given a choice between mammograms or ultrasound, based on the results of this report, would we remotely consider having a mammogram?

My understanding is that if there is a mammogram machine in a clinic, then there is also an ultrasound machine close by. So why not use it? One thing is for sure, you will not get your breasts squashed in the process, there will not be any radiation and the technique is capable of distinguishing between cysts and tumours.

The following report from France appears to confirm the findings of the Cambridge team, telling us that:

> The near-field imaging capability of sonography equipment has recently and markedly improved. High-frequency ultrasonography can improve the specificity of clinically and mammographically detected abnormalities, and helps accurately distinguish benign solid nodules from indeterminate or malignant nodules. The aim of this distinction is to obviate surgical biopsy.[7]

Phrases such as 'ambiguous mammograms' included in the title of this report worry me, whatever the context. My interpretation is that this must place a huge query over the limitations of mammograms and the colossal amount of time wasted by medical staff trying to interpret what is shown on the mammogram they are looking at. Most importantly, the ultrasound technique is clearly capable of pointing out the finer distinctions of different types of lumps.

Ultrasound screening for breast implants

Screening after reconstruction seems to be a subject that is rarely, if ever, discussed – but it appears that you are expected to receive a mammogram just the same. The subject needs to be carefully reviewed when, quite apart from cancer, so many women seek cosmetic breast surgery with implants. A study of women who had undergone breast augmentation was reported in 2002 from Taiwan. A retrospective follow-up study and analysis of diagnostic methods including mammography, sonography, physical examination and aspiration cytology had been conducted on 105 patients who had breast augmentation between 1989 and 2001. Part of the report shows: eight cancer patients were screened with both mammography and ultrasonography, resulting in two tumours being visible on the mammograms and seven tumours diagnosed as cancer by ultrasound. At the end of the detailed report they affirm that sonography is a more useful diagnostic tool than mammography in Taiwanese women who have undergone breast augmentation.[3]

So, if you have implants for whatever reason, the chances are that it would be better to be asking for ultrasound when you next go for screening. Amazingly, the accuracy of physical examination came out equal to that of mammography in this study, reaffirming the fact that it is helpful, whether you do it yourself or a doctor does it. However, advice to women from the UK medical profession in 2004 and publicized on television and in the newspapers was *not* to self-examine as it wasn't thought useful. The report from Taiwan contradicts this advice. When it comes to prevention we clearly need to keep our wits about us and look to our own best interests. Science and health writer Bill Sturgeon points out:

> X-rays are a wonderful medical tool; but, considering the damage they always do, they should not be used on a medical fishing expedition to find disease in otherwise healthy people. There is now a better path to breast cancer screening. If women had available an alternative to mammography, one that detected cancer earlier, harmlessly and with no discomfort, how many would choose it? What would become of all the existing mammogram machines and the people who operate them? I believe we have a widespread conflict of interest, namely the income stream generated by mammography.[4]

Replacing mammogram machines with a safer and more accurate solution is something that we never hear of in the UK, and with new hospitals installing very expensive mammogram machines the future seems firmly stuck in the past. Their replacement would ultimately require expertise and the retraining of those who at present administer mammograms. But playing politics with women's health in order to safeguard jobs and questionable choices, thereby resisting the introduction of better and safer alternative screening, is both sinister and life-threatening. I know that I am not alone in wondering who will actually *implement* these much needed changes.

Other alternatives

Further into my research, I found many tried and tested alternatives to mammograms, some of which have been in existence for many years and approved by the Food and Drugs Administration (FDA) in the USA.

Skin test

Bill Sturgeon tells us that cancer researcher George Springer MD has developed a harmless skin test that can disclose breast cancer using the body's own antigens which can detect cancer up to six years earlier than a mammogram. Sturgeon said, 'Developed years ago, this accurate test remains unavailable to women.'[5]

Electrical current

In America, Dr Leslie Organ pioneered a technique that sends an electrical current through the breast, painlessly and apparently harmlessly to measure speed of flow through the breast. Discrepancies in the flow when comparing both breasts would indicate possible cancer. It is not only cheaper, costing about a third less than the mammogram, but reckoned to be much safer to the extent that it is felt that younger women may benefit from it. Like several new alternatives, it claims to be more accurate than a mammogram in detecting lumps which later turn out to be cancerous. Research continues.[6]

Optical mammography

In the Netherlands, Martin van der Mark of Philips Research in Eindhoven is experimenting with optical mammography. This painless technique involves shining a laser light through the breast. Malignant or benign tumours are detected by analysing the emerging light. It uses apparently insignificant wave lengths which Van der Mark likens to the strength of a normal light bulb. Optical mammography has the capacity to distinguish between benign and malignant tumours but is still in the early stages unlike some of the other methods; nevertheless, this could become another option.

Breath tests

Breath tests are also emerging as a future possibility. This would certainly seem about as low as you could get on the 'invasive procedure' ladder. Research in 2003 showed that a breath test could distinguish between women with breast cancer and healthy volunteers to a sensitivity of 94.1 per cent. When testing women with breast cancer for markers of oxidative stress, it accurately identified these women and showed a negative predictive value (NPV) superior to that of a screening mammogram. It was suggested that this breath test could, potentially, be used as a primary screen for breast cancer.[7]

Blood bio marker testing

Some investigations have found that nuclear matrix protein (NMP), which is not found in healthy women, is present in the blood of women at an early stage of breast cancer and research is being done into blood bio marker testing to detect and monitor women at risk and those already diagnosed with breast cancer. [8]

Scientists at Christie Hospital in Manchester, England, along with researchers at the University of Berne in Switzerland are investigating a similar blood test into two hormones that are present in large amounts in the blood, of which one appears to increase the risk of cancer while the other has been linked to lower cancer risks. A test like this, which could measure the likelihood of a person developing the disease, means that prevention is vital and lifestyle changes to reduce the incidence of cancer need to be researched. [9]

Breast density

Breast density plays a significant role in the interpretation of mammograms. If the breast tissue is very dense it is much more difficult to interpret the mammogram and it is important to understand that breast density is generally greater in some of the black and other ethnic populations, putting them at higher risk of cancer being missed. Moreover, it is said that cancer can appear white, like breast tissue, on a mammogram.

Diet can contribute to increased breast density among both pre-menopausal and post-menopausal women and it is reported that polyunsaturates are associated with increased breast density, thereby endorsing the bad press that has been given to such food products in recent years. Vitamin B12 has also been associated with increased breast density among post-menopausal women, but in cases where women are taking it as a supplement as opposed to the natural intake from food. As is indicated by research, the connection between breast density and dietary factors may be small, but at the same time it is accepted that there could be a connection to the risk of breast cancer. In women of all ages, there appears to be a link between the amount of alcohol we consume and increased breast density. It has been suggested that in post-menopausal women there is a correlation between increased breast density and the consumption of white wine, however, this does not appear to be the same for red wine. All this adds weight to the fact that diet plays an important role in breast health and is good news to the many of us who enjoy a glass of red wine.[10]

Medical infrared thermal imaging (MITI, also called Thermography)

There have already been extensive research and trials with MITI and the published results are tremendously positive. The information given by Dr Nyjon Eccles, BSc. MBBS, PhD, MRCP in his paper 'Thermography – its role in early Breast Cancer Detection and pain monitoring,'[11] is one of the most encouraging yet – the technique having the huge benefit of being radiation free. MITI has also been used for additional diagnostic purposes since the late 1970s.

Dr Eccles informs us that MITI was first used for diagnosis by Lawson in 1957 after discovering that cancerous breast tissue was of a higher temperature than normal breast tissue. As long ago as 1982 the FDA approved this as a screening technique for breast cancer, it showing positive in a minimum of 71 per cent to a maximum of 93 per cent in patients with breast cancer. The figures in Dr Eccles' report show that from 1965 onwards the results have been outstanding. It is clear that this technique has a very high diagnostic accuracy, which he says is 'unparalleled' and 'can clearly identify those who are at high risk'. As both a pharmacologist and a Member of the Royal College of Physicians, his search to find a true pathway in medicine took him to work with Michael Kucera, a medically trained doctor and naturopath, who very successfully treated cancer patients in the former Czech Republic. From there Dr Eccles expanded his search to Spain, India and the USA. In choosing to work with MITI for diagnosis, he believes that cancer can be found much earlier, thereby giving the patient a much better chance of dealing with it.

MITI requires skilled technicians and Dr Eccles says that the patient must follow clear instructions prior to this harmless procedure, such as no alcohol, caffeine, use of lotions, underarm shaving and a few more simple requests which assist in a quality assessment. The thermal imaging camera is remarkably neat, looking a little smaller than a normal television video recorder and posing no threat as it operates by detecting the infrared radiation which is emitted from the body, therefore no X-rays and no sonics! It is very important to make sure that the practitioner has the highest quality of equipment which includes what is known as a '256 part Grey Scale', which shows the vascular patterns in the imaging. In addition, the procedure *must* incorporate a 'cold challenge' whereby at one point in the examination the patient holds an ice pack in each hand in order to send a fight or flight shock to the system as part of a thorough test. At the time of writing, there is a newer MITI system which monitors the breast's response to cold air cooling, the whole scan being reduced to only ten minutes.

Significantly, the procedure gives a much more complete view of the breast with a 360° image available: vital for a woman who has had implants. There is nothing in this test which is invasive to the body, so it *has* to be a huge step forward. Because breast tissue density is immaterial to MITI, women as young as say 20 years old can be tested and, unlike with the mammogram, there is no problem in having an annual check. For those whose results show a possible problem, more frequent screening is advised. It is especially valuable, not only because it can predict so far ahead – six years or more is not unusual – but also because it is safe for women of all ages. Dr Eccles points out that some reports have accused MITI of being wrong, showing the thermal imaging as 'positive' when the mammogram showed 'negative'. In many of these cases, some five to ten years later, breast cancer has shown up exactly on the spot indicated by the MITI.

Finding breast cancer early

Predicting far ahead means that a breast cancer almost the size of a pinprick could be detected long before it becomes a tumour and, as explained earlier, we know that the tumour usually arrives several years after its initial manifestation in the body (*see* page 50). Now, with this vital, early information, it has to be a much more straightforward task to unravel what is only the start of a problem rather than dealing with an advanced tumour years down the line. This could be the beginning of the end of breast surgery. As Dr Eccles said to me, it would then be a case of:

> … placing those women with positive findings into the appropriate lifestyle modification and treatment model which may be able to prevent or minimize not only cancer, but all breast disease … there is no reason to simply 'wait and see' any longer … If caught early, cancer is a treatable disease.[12]

We need it immediately, so why do the medical profession, the NHS and the UK government not abandon mammograms now? Why wait, when this technique was approved by the FDA in 1982? How do you give this 'old news' to my young friend Kiran who was told that the original diagnosis of a cyst was found, three years later, to be incorrect and actually it was breast cancer?

The role of prevention

In 2001, the UK government set up a review body, headed by Derek Wanless, to assess the long-term resource requirements for the NHS. Entitled 'Securing Our Future Good Health', the Wanless report called for prevention and it has been suggested that prevention is the 'new cure'. But in reality this is nothing new. The idea that the function of medical carers is to help people to help themselves has been around since Hippocrates. Apparently the reason for this 'new-found' approach is to stem the rising rates of diabetes, sexual infection and the results of alcohol abuse. Well aware that the NHS is not able to cope with escalating demands, either in the present or in the future, a decision has been made to begin a programme of prevention.

The prevention of breast cancer by mammogram screening is clearly not in our best interests and it is up to us all – men and women – to call for the necessary changes, so that by demanding non-damaging breast screening we get what we rightly deserve: the best technology *and prevention*. If a potential cancer can be identified through MITI or other non-invasive forms of screening five or six years before the tumour develops, it would be totally impractical – indeed, inconceivable – to send the patient away to wait until such time as the tumour arrives and surgery becomes the only option. Something *has* to be done and can be done to help prevent it happening in the meantime. It is quite evident that science has the resources that we need to help us. All of us are waiting for this help to be allowed into our lives.

15 Menopause – Balancing the System

I want to know if you can live with failure, yours and mine, and still stand on the edge of the lake and shout to the silver of the full moon, 'Yes!'

Oriah Mountain Dreamer [1]

Self-confidence

The menopause is indeed a strange time in a woman's life; in general our society has little time for it. Information is available on the physical aspects of menopause, but the wisdom of the older woman is afforded little respect. At this crucial time in their lives, youth is no longer there to ease the journey and women seem to be all too easily herded into the limited categories of being middle-aged, elderly and old.

Perhaps one of the most important keys to the menopause is to be able to understand yourself, to consciously be able to recognize your strengths and weaknesses and with an open mind stay true to yourself. I remember having a conversation some years ago with a woman in her mid-forties who was working as a sales assistant in a large retail clothing store. The subject was middle-aged women and she said how disturbing she found it that so many of these women seemed uncertain and lacking in confidence, needing advice and reassurance in their choice of clothing. It left me wondering just how many middle-aged women really do lack confidence, and, if this is the case, why?

Attitude of the media

The UK pop industry is driven by money and aimed at teenagers – 13 to 14 year olds. In Europe, however, a wide variety of popular music and performances by older artists of both sexes are commonplace, whilst in the US there is a buoyant music market for those over 40. Somehow in the UK our media-driven existence seems to refer only to the disadvantages of getting older, and reinforces the idea of young girls being the most desirable. Taking a look at the nation's psyche, writer Lauren Booth observed that Jordan – whose physical attributes make her a UK glamour model – was Britain's most searched-for female on the Internet in 2004. If it wasn't for occasional praise being given to middle-aged actresses such as our own Helen Mirren, you might think that attractive, intelligent women in this age group didn't exist, the very British trait of self-destruct, the 'damned if you do, damned if you don't' attitude seeming to dampen any possible idea that we should celebrate the older woman. An article in the *Sunday Times Style Magazine* criticizing older women for trying to look young by dyeing their hair blonde seemed an extraordinary assault.[2] Was it tongue in cheek? Of course! The British are good at that: it was another joke at the expense of older women. As my hairdresser succinctly put it, 'Are you supposed to roll over and die?' No wonder that the French, Italians and Germans are often mystified by the attitude of our press and media who appear to collude in undermining us. This is a time when women should be free, accountable only to themselves and listened to for the wisdom they might have to offer.

Changing role

Small wonder then that British middle-aged women in particular often question their role and where they belong in society. At the menopause, a woman's life has a different set of stresses and strains from those it had when her children were younger. Soon it will no longer be possible for women to receive a state pension at 60. They will have to wait until 65, and yet the menopause cannot be delayed. Financially many women still need to continue to bring in an income, whether married or single, whilst others see the window of freedom from raising a family slip away as our economy creates difficulties for those children, now grown up, who have just left full-time education. Many young people go off to university, only to return to the family home three or four years later because they are unable to finance their own accommodation. This return home, which occurs just at the time when a young person would really prefer to be independent and living elsewhere, gives rise to a woman appearing to take on the role of mother once again.

Middle age should be a time of self-evaluation in order for people to set a new, creative pathway for the future and growing older. Most women instinctively know how to handle things, whether through bringing up families or through experience and responsibilities in the workplace. Their life experience has enabled them to adjust to others' agendas, but now, it is time for change. It is the time when a woman must guard the right to say 'no' to excessive demands and be supported in doing so.

Strained physical resources

Making a stand requires utilizing both physical and mental resources. At a physical level, it is quite common for women to feel more easily tired and generally not at one with themselves as changes in the body gather momentum and the imbalance of hormones has the potential to cause problems. It is still unclear why some women pass through this transition without any difficulty, as if the menopause had never happened, whilst the experience of others varies from the odd night sweat to hot flashes that seem relentless around the clock. If nothing else, it indicates how very much the menopause is an individual journey, with each woman reacting slightly differently as her body moves through the subtle changes in hormone levels as the hormones shift their principal production from the ovaries to the adrenals.

Many years of working under stress will make depletion worse at the menopause, and when we feel ill the dangerous habit of 'keeping going' – something that happens all too often to both men and women of all ages – puts a huge overload on the immune system. Perhaps one of the explanations for the proliferation of the 'diseases of modern civilization' is the fact that our modern way of life has conditioned us to believe that the 'right' course of action when we are ill is to take a pill and carry on regardless. Each person differs in how their system will cope with this assault and it is something we cannot anticipate. Suppression is dangerous: to be able to submit to a fever, go to bed and sweat it out is, as we already know, the healthy solution. There are cases recognized by doctors, where, for no accountable reason, a cancer patient has gone into a state of fever as a result of some infection, and come out of it free from cancer. Cancer cells do not like heat and so a natural fever is a positive advantage, but not so likely to happen when the immune system is depressed. Allowing ourselves the time to be ill is an essential ingredient in maintaining health at the menopause.

A delicate balance

If you are feeling unduly tired, stressed or just concerned about your health at this time, then it is important to seek help. In addition to having standard blood tests, research indicates that it might be wise to keep a check on hormone, vitamin and mineral levels as a prevention against possible later disease, including breast cancer. Scientific evidence increasingly suggests that it is the delicate balance of all the physical aspects of health, plus the avoidance of stress, and most importantly, maintaining a happy, balanced life, that will steer a good course through the menopausal years. It also indicates that a very fine margin may exist between a woman getting breast cancer or not. Some doctors believe that, almost without exception, women with breast cancer have lower levels of thyroid function, melatonin and adrenaline. Until recently, there has been little interest in these facts which are now gradually being recognized as significant. As the work of Dr Fryda shows, it is important that when depletions are found, action is taken to rectify the problems and then monitored, as very often the body will rebalance itself with encouragement.

Breast cancer – a menopause overload

One side effect of a depleted physical system is to take the easy route and just go with the flow, suppressing your own stronger feelings, beliefs and intuition – a treacherous path to take as this also consumes considerable amounts of energy, contributing further to the general depletion of energy levels affecting the immune system and facilitating the onset of disease. By the time the menopause arrives, the energy that may previously have been ready to stand up and deal with all events can be lacking. On the other hand, with good energy available, you may have sensibly decided that you have reached a point where it is necessary to become rather more discriminating about your life choices. However, if you have breast cancer at this time, it becomes a minefield, and taking a stand calls on far greater resources than it would have done before. With the likelihood of prescribed surgery, radiotherapy and/or chemotherapy, it is not surprising that a woman can become dangerously stressed. On top of all this there will be further hormonal upset, as it is very likely that she will lose lymph nodes and part, or all, of her breast. The possible loss of her hair will be a further blow to her femininity.

It does not take much to understand the enormous trauma and loss of a sense of self that breast cancer – plus the menopause – brings with it. Putting a brave face on this alone requires huge energy, just when you have so little to fall back on, and sadly, it is happening to so many of us. It is unlikely at this time of change that regaining 'normality' is going to happen speedily; it requires huge commitment, sensitivity and understanding, not only from the woman, but also from her family and those close to her. Following the hospital treatment, many of the tests and complementary therapies vital to regaining balanced and good health will have to be found outside the conventional health system, which takes time, patience and money. Be prepared to try several routes as this is where reliance on your own intuition, communication with other understanding women, sympathetic practitioners and therapists, all become essential in order to find the best solutions to personal problems. With the proper help and good people around you, it is possible to become strong and healthy again.

Chemotherapy, tamoxifen and the menopause

The medical profession acknowledges that chemotherapy aggravates menopausal symptoms, and the effectiveness of this treatment is queried by many doctors who recognize the importance of rebalancing the hormones at this stage of a woman's life. Those women who receive chemotherapy will often be left with a whole collection of problems to sort out, and one of the biggest difficulties for them is to understand if a newly arising problem is a menopausal one or something to do with the cancer. It is a continual worry, and unless a woman has the help of an exception- ally good, understanding doctor, she will often be left to sort out these problems by herself. Tamoxifen alone can create menopausal symptoms in younger women as well as those of menopausal age and this can be very distressing, the oestrogen levels dropping because of the treatment and causing confusion to a woman as she tries to regain her health.

There are now many more products available to help deal with menopausal problems. It seems to be very much trial and error and what suits one doesn't always suit another. Some of the home-opathic products are gentler on the system and, like other products for the menopause, they may take some weeks to have a full effect. It is also worth investigating companies who specialize in women's health. Some of these produce balancing endocrine tonics suitable for the menopause.[3] There are numerous preparations readily available for period and menopausal problems, which do not involve harmful man-made hormones. Leslie Kenton gives a most comprehensive list of such alternatives in *Passage to Power* but, if you have breast cancer and feel uncertain about which ones are safe to use, consult a practitioner with an interest in women's health and complementary medicine.

Good health

In his book *A Cancer Therapy*, Dr Max Gerson says:

> A normal body has the capacity to keep all cells
> functioning properly. It prevents any abnormal
> transformation and growth. Therefore, the natural task of
> a cancer therapy is to bring the body back to that normal
> physiology, or as near to it as possible. The next task is to
> keep the physiology of the metabolism in that natural
> equilibrium.

It is this natural equilibrium, the recognition of it and our ability to keep an eye on it that is vital; there is a real need for us to be active in preserving our health. The list of essentials might be simply outlined as:

- Diet and self-nurture
- Exercise

- Avoidance of a stressful lifestyle
- Creativity. Anything outside yourself that draws on inspiration for both work and play.

Cancer is negative creativity, so self-esteem and the determination to get the best from life will be a very positive step, both physically and psychologically. It seems wise to avoid being overstressed and above all to keep a balance, so don't push yourself when it is obvious you need to take it easy. Often people who have overcome cancer have also overcome the lack of creativity in their lives, opening up time for interests that previously they would not have considered. These new creative challenges bring a good energy – it could even be described as a 'good stress' – the physical benefits arising from these activities being vital to good health. It is a time to experiment and choose what suits you, closing the door on any activity which becomes a drain on your energies. The menopause requires us to make a stand, call the shots, and demand the best for ourselves, both outwardly and inwardly.

16 Breast Care, Risks and Prevention

Oestrogens, the contraceptive pill and antibiotics

It is now believed that part of the breast cancer problem is due to us being exposed to oestrogens over a longer period of our lives. Women with early menopause apparently have less danger of getting breast cancer, whilst those who have an early onset of menstruation have almost twice the risk. In an article titled 'Breast Cancer – A Preventable Disease', Dr Samuel Epstein and David Steinman tell us that oestrogen-dependent cancer, particularly among post-menopausal women, increased by 130 per cent from the mid-1970s to mid-1980. Non-oestrogen cancer increased in that period by 27 per cent.[1] There is much information available on the dangers of artificial oestrogens caused by chemicals and pharmaceuticals to support this. (*See* chapter 13, Our Environment)

The contraceptive pill leaves women vulnerable, and the more recent 'low-dose' pill, with less artificial oestrogen and progesterone, which was initially thought to be less harmful, is now proving to be a problem as women are more likely to believe the low-dose pill to be safer and consequently use it for longer periods of time. In 1995, *The Journal of the National Cancer Institute* reported that the use of contraceptive pills can increase the chances of breast cancer by 30 per cent after only a few months. The risk doubled after using it for ten years or more. The added problem of a lack of fertility has also been caused by the pill: women over 35 who had been taking it took two and a half times longer to become pregnant than those who had not. This problem appears to be greater in the obese and those with irregular periods. With this kind of information at hand, it is easy to foresee the potentially catastrophic consequences of very young girls being given oral contraceptives and hormone contraceptive implants or injections.

Certain antibiotics, antidepressants and cholesterol-reducing drugs are also said to cause cancer later on. A recent study by Christine Velicer at the Department of Epidemiology at the University of Washington, Seattle, added support to the issue, confirming the alarming fact that women who frequently use antibiotics such as penicillin, increase their breast cancer risk by as much as 50 per cent. Some women in the study were as young as 19, and even antibiotics for acne seem to increase the chances of breast cancer later. Trying to find a reason for this, some specialists thought it likely that suppressing the chronic inflammation could open up the possibility for tumours to develop. It appears that all classes of antibiotics increase the risk.[2] (*See also* chapters 12 and 13.)

Benefits of breastfeeding

Research indicates that women who breastfeed several children stand a far better chance of avoiding breast cancer than those who don't. Breast tissue is very sensitive to environmental carcinogens between the onset of menstruation up to the first pregnancy, whilst mature breast cells – those after pregnancy – are 50 per cent less susceptible to cancer caused by environmental factors. It would appear that the more babies you have, the less your risk of breast cancer caused by environmental agents, and breastfeeding appears to lower the level of carcinogens in the breast and in the body fat.

Breast cysts

Many women are at a disadvantage by having a tendency to develop cysts or what are often described as 'lumpy' breasts. Whatever your age, it is a common problem and bound to cause worry, as it can be difficult to know whether they are just harmless cysts or not. The problem at the menopause is that if you have a history of cysts going back many years, you become vulnerable to the illogical assumption by some doctors that all breast lumps you present are cysts. At the beginning of March 2004, both newspapers and television were telling us that self-examination of the breasts for cancer was harmful – a seemingly ludicrous and dangerous guideline. As you may remember from chapter 14, 'Alternatives to Mammograms' self-examination is proven to be helpful (*see* page 182).

Cysts: a natural cure

I had a benign cyst under my armpit for ten years, which would become larger around the time of a period. My GP explained that it was not a problem, as the cyst was a sebaceous one, just under the skin rather than in the armpit. However, it was still affected by the monthly cycle, becoming larger and more tender during that time. When I changed from using a standard deodorant, to a natural one, the whole thing completely disappeared, never to return. It would have been very useful to have had guidance from my GP instead of eventually solving the problem myself. Experiences of many friends and colleagues indicate that it is often the luck of the draw as to how informed and helpful your GP is concerning environmental issues and women's health.

Prevention of breast cysts

How then can we best look after our breasts, whilst abandoning potentially harmful cosmetic products? It seems that we can do things to not only change breast density by diet, but also to help ourselves with the problem of cysts through supplements. Celia Wright tells us that vitamin E appears to be protective to breasts. A dose of vitamin E-200iu, given to women by Dr Abrams at Boston University School of Medicine in 1965, showed a 65 per cent reduction in cyst size. In 1978, Dr London at the Sinai Hospital, Baltimore, found an overall response of 85 per cent with higher doses of 600iu, noting that if a woman were to respond she would do so within two menstrual cycles.[3]

Dr Peter Minton, at Ohio State University College of Medicine, found that fibrocystic breasts contained greater levels of cyclic nucleotides, chemicals which stimulate cell growth. As a possible culprit, he queried certain food chemicals called methylxanthines, which are known to block nucleotide breakdown. His results were quite dramatic. Out of 45 women, 37 had complete resolution of their cysts within two to six months, 7 reported less discomfort and only one experienced no change. Methylxanthines are found in caffeine – in cola drinks, chocolate, tea and coffee for example. None of these reports are new, but many women are still unaware of the benefits that they might gain from acting on their results.[4]

Cysts and oestrogen dominance

American Dr John Lee was a pioneer in understanding oestrogen dominance and expressed the view that oestrogen dominance is the cause of fibrocystic breasts. Oestrogen tends to encourage cell division whereas progesterone reduces this effect. So if there is a lack of progesterone, the breast cells may divide excessively. It seems that it is not uncommon for women over 35 to fail to ovulate each month despite having periods – possibly caused by chemical pollution. The result of this can be lumpy cysts. Lee advocates the use of natural progesterone to revert the breast to normal. There are several schools of thought on the use of natural progesterone cream, of which there are many types, so it is important to look into it and ask for expert advice if you are thinking of using it.[5]

Cysts: a cure with melatonin

Robert Jacobs, a leading naturopath working in London and Los Angeles, found that in one of his patients a persistent breast lump, which was thought to be a cyst, disappeared after three months of her taking a melatonin supplement. More research has been done recently, showing that melatonin has great powers as an antioxidant as well as a hormone regulator.

Melatonin

Melatonin is the hormone that kicks in at night when the body is ready to sleep. Melatonin's opposite, as it were, is seratonin, the hormone that keeps us alert during the daylight hours. It is essential that we get proper sleep for the immune system to work well and for this to happen the body requires an adequate melatonin level. At certain times, we can have our sleep disrupted for a variety of reasons and many of us have lived through being kept awake, often night after night, with a child or dependant who is unwell. At the menopause, sleeping can often be particularly difficult and it appears that there is a natural drop in melatonin levels around the age of 50, according to research in the UK by Roger Coghill. His tests show that women with breast cancer may have as little as 10 per cent of the normal levels of melatonin, and research into night-shift workers shows them to be more susceptible than most to this problem.[6]

Lack of melatonin induced by stress

Thomas Saunders gives a description of the valuable role of melatonin in his book, *The Boiled Frog Syndrome*:

> The release of vital secretions from the endocrine glands
> is controlled by the brainwave patterns. When we feel

drowsy our electrical brainwave patterns change from beta – the normal level when we are awake – to alpha. As we fall asleep, begin dreaming and then move to the deeper hypnotic and psychic subconscious experiences, so the electrical pulse rate changes further to delta and gamma frequency levels that control the release of essential secretions from other endocrine glands. Relatively weak shifts in the strength of natural electromagnetic fields radiating from the Earth and outer space, or from artificially generated electromagnetic fields, can set up interference patterns with the brain's minute electrical wave activity. Such disturbance to the brain's release mechanism of the endocrine secretions affects our biological rhythms, mood swings, stress levels and reproduction cycles, and depletes our immune system. Any form of sleep deprivation, such as sleeping in a room which is not dark, will suppress the production of melatonin resulting in clinical depression or non-clinical depression such as jet lag. Shift work can have the same effect. When we are seriously ill, part of nature's cure is to keep us asleep for long periods to allow melatonin and other secretions to replenish and boost the immune system … Our immune system also depends on melatonin to regulate the levels of the hormone oestrogen, which is linked to breast cancer. Artificial light, jet lag and shift work (including flight crews) disrupts the production of melatonin.[7]

We clearly need to protect our immediate environment not only for ourselves, but also for the very young as they would benefit from having a dark bedroom rather than artificial light through the night.

Dangers for shift workers

The possible indication of a relationship between shift work and breast cancer was published in two articles in the *Journal of the National Cancer Institute* in the United States where it was suggested that the effect of altered light exposure at night on the levels of melatonin or other hormones in the body might increase the risk of breast cancer. Following the publication of this research in the UK, the Health and Safety Executive (HSE) commissioned Professor Anthony Swerdlow, a leading epidemiologist at the Institute of Cancer Research to investigate. Professor Swerdlow's subsequent report, *Shiftwork and breast cancer: A critical review of the epidemiological evidence* concluded, 'Overall, the evidence for an association is appreciable, but not definitive' and that 'further epidemiological research is needed to clarify the relationship.'[8] Sandra Caldwell, co-director of policy at the HSE was quick to play down the possible association with breast cancer, saying, 'The review suggests that so far epidemiological research is inconclusive about the link between breast cancer risk and shift work, if any, and further research will be necessary to clarify the relation.' Looking ahead, it appears that a group of international and national medical experts will assemble to decide how the research can progress. Caldwell pointed out the difficulties of identifying how shift work, especially extended night shifts, could be involved in breast cancer as the risks from genetics, the environment and behaviour complicate the issue.[9] Will it be another case of the buck being passed, research having created a picture which looks too complex to deal with? Or, just maybe, after a long time and many committees, will there be some sort of a conclusion?

Balancing hormones

Hormones have been frequently suspected of playing a part in the possible cause of breast cancer, making reasonable an association with the menopause when the hormones are changing and the ovaries are no longer producing the sex hormones, their production now moving to the adrenals, liver and fat cells. The study of hormones and their behaviour – including oestrogen, progesterone, melatonin, adrenal androgen performance and the thyroid – in order to provide some sort of evidence of the role they might play in breast cancer has gone on for many years without reaching any definite conclusion, but it is still thought that there may be some link.[10]

Both our adrenal levels and our adrenal-vitamin C levels lower with age. Beta-carotene is the major carotenoid in the adrenal glands, so, as mentioned earlier, carrot juice provides a good source of beta-carotene (see page 155). Clearly, healthy adrenal and hormone functions are reliant on each other, so it is crucial to keep them both in the best possible condition.[11] The authors of this research reinforce the necessity of keeping a delicate balance telling us, 'The goal of the treatment is to relieve symptoms of hormone deficiency and achieve near-normal blood hormone levels.' The delicate balance of our system is a recurring theme in women's health.

The adrenal gland and immune function are said to be protected by vitamin E. Selenium assists the process as an anti-oxidant, as does zinc. Magnesium is vital in keeping the balance and particularly needs maintaining around the menopause, working in conjunction with calcium to prevent osteoporosis and also helping cells to shift hormones around the body. Dr B Durrant-Peatfield in his article in the *ICM Journal* suggests that we need 450mg of magnesium a day, and tells us that in 1997 the National Academy of Sciences in the USA confirmed that most Americans are magnesium deficient as a result of consuming overprocessed food and drink.[12] Anna Cocilovo, a complementary practitioner, points out that magnesium is very important when we are looking into stress. She tells us that if we are stressed, our cells can become depleted of magnesium and if we release our stress, the body resumes a normal balance once again. By raising our levels of magnesium, we also help relieve the stress. She emphasizes the need for magnesium in order for the body to properly absorb calcium and like many practitioners she also encourages taking a supplement to help provide essential fatty acids.[13]

All information about minerals and vitamins and how they interact is important to consider in keeping healthy. It is good to know that by having a generous intake of varied, natural food – particularly fruits and vegetables – we can increase our capacity to ward off so many degenerative health problems, at the same time helping the body to maintain a healthy balance.

Whatever a woman's age, the balancing of hormones is of prime importance, as if this is ignored, it gives rise to all kinds of debilitating symptoms. With the disturbing revelations about hormone replacement therapy and the contraceptive pill, we are now looking for a more natural method of dealing with problems in both young and menopausal women. There are many practitioners and doctors who are beginning to be much more aware of alternative ways to help find a solution, and an increasing amount of information is available on the subject.

Homeopathy

Many people may not be aware that it is possible to deal with maintaining healthy breast tissue and clearing cysts with homeopathy. Homeopathy has always been very important to me as a remedy for general family ailments and after my treatment in Germany I found it more valuable than ever (*see* page 77). Should you be in any doubt about the merits of homeopathy, the *British Medical Journal* published a very favourable summary of research showing the effectiveness of homeopathy in the treatment of disease. The authors were medical school professors who were asked by the Dutch government to review the existing research.[14]

Other therapies

Acupuncture, reflexology, cranial osteopathy, massage, meditation, NLP and psychotherapy are just some of the therapies that have an important role to play. You may find that one particular therapy is the most beneficial – again, follow your gut feelings. My reflexology sessions with Tony Porter in London gave support to the adrenal regeneration I had received in Germany, whilst Saied Shahsavari at the Holistic Health Clinic in north London, who is highly qualified in many alternative therapies, gave lymph-drainage massage to clear the system of stagnation and toxins after I was tumour-free and recovered. It is generally believed that body massage is not good until the cancer has been cleared, otherwise you are vulnerable to the toxins being spread around the system. Saied uses both the traditional and new methods of lymph drainage in combination, the end result of this gentle massage being a wonderfully destressed body with the lymph glands prompted into action. Check out your local library, complementary therapists and women's groups in your area for information.

Diet

Concerning diet, we already know that 'differences in breast density across all levels of dietary factors were small in magnitude but may have implications for breast cancer risk' (*see* page 185). So those doctors who still believe that you can eat whatever you want, as there is not sufficient evidence to the contrary, are not helping the cause, whilst at the same time contradicting the fact that the Cancer Prevention Research Trust has acknowledged the association of diet and the prevention of cancer for many years. Their recent report in *Cancer Prevention and Health News* highlighted the possible implications in the case of breast cancer, which we cannot afford to overlook. Considering how sophisticated the body is, it would seem reasonable that delicate balancing is essential at every level.[15]

Avoid processed foods

Most of the food we can buy has added preservatives and flavour enhancers. As I mentioned earlier, it was a vital part of my programme to eat organically and drink at least a litre and a half of water a day. The way food is processed in crucial to our understanding of how to eat for health. Foods such as sausages, some ready-cooked cold meats and smoked fish are just a few that can often be quite heavily processed and may contain large amounts of preservatives. Reports on the connection between some sugar substitutes and cancer remind us of the need to be watchful. Always read the small print.

Eat wholegrain and fresh

Try to establish a routine of eating wholly organic, wholegrain and fresh. This, plus juicing, provides great nutrition and a healthy diet. There is a wealth of recipe books in this growing market, the main requirement being a bit of time to put your imagination into action in the kitchen. The more you submerge yourself in it, the easier it becomes to experiment and adapt certain good, basic recipes to suit your needs and tastes. A general rule of thumb seems to be that if you can eat around 80 per cent organic, you are doing well. This seems reasonable without being manically rigid! There is also available an increasing selection of ready-prepared sauces and soups which are organic, fresh and free from additives – a great help when pressed for time.

Be empowered

Again, if you are in any in doubt, it might be very worth your while to get an analysis of the state of your mineral, vitamin and hormone levels, which can be done easily as many laboratories run these tests; at least it will be a baseline to start from. Supplementing the diet with high-quality natural food nutrition supplements allows the body to balance itself. These are well worth looking into as it seems they are preferable to using lots of over-the-counter vitamin supplements. All these factors need to be taken into account if you want to do the best for your health and build up a barrier between yourself and illness. Remember that a woman's hormonal system is highly sophisticated and individual. The onset of menarche, taking the Pill, having babies and the menopause are all times of major change and fluctuation. Give yourself the best that you can find in every way. Be intelligent about it, and don't allow your system to be assaulted with a sledgehammer of medication when it is feeling under par. Proceed the feminine way, with flexibility, letting your own body guide you. If you need help, whatever your age, search for the person who has empathy and tries to really understand you and your needs. When taking responsibility for your health, you deserve the best you can find.

PART FOUR

Getting to the Heart of Health

We are sound. The question of what we allow to be transmitted from ourselves to others, and what we allow to enter our own systems is everyone's privilege to decide.

Herbert Whone

Mindful choosing of friends and lovers, not to mention teachers, is critical to remaining conscious, remaining intuitive, remaining in charge of the fiery light that sees and knows.

Clarissa Pinkola Estés

17 A Holistic View

Pythagoras held the key to harmony as we know it today. It was through him that Hippocrates was able to understand that the health of a human being relies on the wholeness of body, mind and spirit residing in us in harmony. Originally 'science' and 'spirituality' were not separated as they are today, and it is this separation that has resulted in our loss of vision of our potential harmonious wholeness of being. The subsequent ever-narrower specialization of the sciences has culminated in a tunnel vision that increasingly ignores 'the whole'. This tunnel vision is prevalent among those scientists who, being neither creative nor original thinkers, slavishly follow the consensus view. Seeing that we were being led down these confining pathways to our detriment, T S Eliot succinctly asked in his poem, *The Rock*:

> *Where is the life we have lost in living?*
>
> *Where is the wisdom we have lost in knowledge?*
>
> *Where is the knowledge we have lost in information?*

The need for a holistic approach in medicine and music

The current treatment of breast cancer appears to be the product of tunnel vision, with the medical establishment basing its methods of diagnosis and treatment on a general pattern which is either empirical or rationalistic in outlook, but has very little place in the holistic health of the individual. With this kind of attitude, what is going on at the root is of no concern. Here there are parallels to be drawn with inadequate vocal teaching, whereby a voice is forced to conform to a preconceived 'suitable' sound – the equivalent of conforming to a set of physical symptoms. Convinced that bodies (and voices) are all similar, it is not deemed necessary by the medical establishment to search any deeper, and so routine, standard procedures are followed in the belief that these will suffice. The suggestion that something is glaringly amiss at a deeper level is brushed aside with the belief that, given time and by adhering to the normal course of action, all will be well. This is not being in touch with reality.

In the case of the singer continuing obliviously along this pathway towards the 'suitable' sound with a false sense of security, he or she eventually receives a wake-up call when they are devastated to find that their public performances meet with a lukewarm reception from the critics, whilst their family and friends can only support them in their anguish and subsequent lack of employment. For a personal parallel to this in medicine, I need only look back on my early, missed diagnosis, where it appeared to be more important for some members of the medical establishment to provide me with a false sense of security.

Compromise and choice

Compromise is something that we all have to deal with in our lives, but it should not be the basis of our health services. GPs cannot possibly work to the best of their abilities with only five minutes allocated to every patient. Doctors appear to be at the mercy of the NHS, government and bureaucracy, with the NHS now seeking help from private hospitals to cope with its own backlog of patients, further ensuring that private medicine becomes merely another arm of the NHS. If we could choose our own doctors, the last thing we would want is to have to settle for second best. Many doctors have already left the NHS, unable to compromise their standards with the system, in the same way that many of our scientists have left the country to work in a freer environment. Those scientists who retain a holistic vision often find that because their work (both practical and theoretical) does not fit into the consensus view they are ostracized by the mainstream scientific establishment – i.e. they rock the boat. The consequent loss to both the health service and to us, the patients, is immeasurable.[1]

I receive telephone calls from students from time to time, seeking advice in choosing a teacher. Naturally I listen to them carefully, but as I may never speak with many of them again, I always emphasize that whoever they choose, the tuition must feel right, there should be no discomfort either physically or mentally and the work should follow the natural laws of the body. If this is the case, and they are having a diligent, joyful and fulfilling experience with a teacher, then obviously they should stay and learn. If not, don't waste time – move on.

Science, art and the voice

Where the science of the voice is concerned, medical textbooks provide the information and diagrams necessary for gaining an understanding of the mechanism of the vocal chords and other relevant parts of the body that directly play a role in the making of sound. Rudolf Steiner, the eminent mystic and scientist (1861–1925), was able to calculate through his deep understanding and knowledge of anatomy that the human voice has available a basic range of three octaves, which can be extended further. Steiner saw no barriers between art and science other than those that we create for ourselves, and he believed that the ultimate creation emanated from 'the whole' and could only be achieved by a holistic approach. The voice is the only musical instrument 'inside' us and not external to our body, which makes it easier to access in some ways, but also more difficult to be objective about it. Neither a purely scientific and technical approach, nor a purely artistic approach, would produce the beauty of sound that we seek; it would be quite unthinkable for either a singer or an instrumentalist to perform in such an isolated manner.

The job of the teacher

Conventional teaching methods tend to work backwards, continually correcting that which is wrong. Acknowledging that there *are* things that can be wrong – just as there are when we are ill – the return to wholeness demands a much more positive approach, unravelling the present 'wrong' situation whilst simultaneously reinforcing the good and pointing out how this 'good' has been achieved. For me, this is a very necessary part of the process to restore either a good voice or good health.

No magic bullet

The journey to find a person's true voice takes place physically as well as mentally, psychologically and spiritually. It cannot be short-circuited by a magic bullet. If it could, the individual would neither deepen their understanding of their voice nor learn how to prevent any problems that might occur in the future. Moreover, a quick-fix solution would not reveal their greater creative potential. As in medicine, the fine-tuning ability of the practitioner and the willingness to be creative regarding the health of the patient based on knowledge, sensitivity and understanding, is crucial. In pursuit of the best, the ego of the doctor or teacher has to be pushed aside and, as Dr Fryda puts it, a willingness to 'get under the skin and connect with the soul of the patient' becomes vital in order to truly understand those you are trying to help.

Insight is the key

I remember a young woman doctor saying that her father, also a doctor, had emphasized that above all, she must listen extremely carefully to her patients, because by listening she would find the answers she needed. The same applies in my own work as I search for clues about the person in front of me. By listening carefully, I can find vast amounts of information to guide my understanding of the singer, and gain valuable insights into what makes him or her tick, how they live, what they expect, their fears, how they see themselves and so on.

No good teacher 'creates' a voice, but rather empowers the student to reveal their own beauty. The minute you notice them forging ahead, the more subtly and delicately you need to fine-tune and nudge them into the further unfolding of their talent.

The rigid approach

The results of bad teaching are as obvious as the results of badly applied medicine. In the introduction to *Singing and the Etheric Tone*, Dina Soresi Winter says:

> ... singers with initially good voices emerged [from rigid tuition] in desperation from these vocal studios ... Some sought their own paths and found the key which led them to their own individual singing freedom. Birgit Nilsson, the great Swedish soprano, was one who did ... Singing ... connects us with our divine, spiritual origins. [2]

The similarly rigid approach that we receive with the 'one cure for all' in medicine is always going to incite certain instinctive individuals, rather like the singers just mentioned, to search for a cure elsewhere. This combination of intuition and individuality is something that the medical profession very often condemns or refuses to recognize, particularly in the case of cancer. It may not always be a success, but these individuals have made it their own responsibility to find a pathway to a more sensitive, understanding and, in some cases, an infinitely more successful and healthy outcome than would otherwise have been achieved had they remained with the rigid 'one cure for all' approach.

Like the treatment I underwent with Dr Fryda for the cancer, the problem is unravelled by a process of gently restoring the body to its proper function and subsequent healthy use. It is the same principle – a restorative/reversal process – that Roger Coghill is searching for in the suppressed work of Koch (*see* page 157).

After repair – prevention

The end result of the process will be both restorative and preventative which, as far as the singer is concerned, is paramount – as it is useless to restore the voice and then sing your way back into trouble by ignoring what caused the problem in the first place. Few cancer patients who follow the conventional route of cut, poison and burn can be entirely sure that the disease will not recur, because the aim of the treatment has been to 'fix' the symptoms. As with the singer who is empowered by the knowledge that he or she can now maintain a healthy voice, thereby opening up the opportunity for boundless creativity, the cancer patient requires a course of treatment that not only restores the whole body, but also empowers them with an understanding necessary to maintain good health, both now and in the future – even to the extent that they become healthier than before.

Music, the healer

We are just beginning to realize the enormous potential of what is referred to as 'vibrational medicine', often spoken of as the medicine of the future and already evident in ultrasound. It is not a new discovery. Sound has always been used to heal, and the amazing healing qualities of music have been deeply explored in the 20th century by Dr Roberto Assagioli, founder of psychosynthesis, and Dr Alfred Tomatis who created Audio-Psycho-Phonology (APP), which deals with the way we listen.[3] The discovery by Tomatis that listening problems are the root cause of many learning problems has led to healing work with autism, dyslexia, attention deficit disorders and many learning-related problems.[4] I recall reading the story of two French women with breast cancer, who attempted to heal themselves by chanting for two or three hours a day for three months under the supervision of a doctor and a nun whose research indicated that chanting to the correct vibrations might well heal their cancer. Both women had said they would have an operation for the breast cancer after the experiment, perhaps not expecting the chanting to significantly reduce the size of the lumps in their breasts. The results were astonishing: one of the women no longer required surgery, and the other found the lump so much reduced that the surgeon was able to perform a successful lumpectomy, which was made all the easier because the lump had become completely encased thereby protecting her from any possible metastases. I never heard any more of this remarkable story, perhaps because the successful treatment involved time and not money! It surely has to be the most magical and gentle approach possible: non-toxic, no bullets of destruction and devoid of any side effects. It is a wonderful example of music balancing body and soul and also healing the 'troubled breast'. Through sound these women found the whole; the golden key to their self-healing ability, inner peace and harmony.

18 Medical Neuro-Linguistic Programming (NLP)

I knew very little about Neuro-Linguistic Programming before deciding that it might be a tool to help my recovery. Previous experiences and my awareness through music and teaching had shown me how the mind can touch depths and emotions, which in turn trigger a bodily response. In a similar manner, NLP, with its acceptance of the importance of the mind body connection, seemed to suggest that it could be a fast track to regaining my health, and that I would feel as if I had some control over my recovery – something very important to me. After a brief search, it was suggested that I contact Garner Thomson, one of the world's leading authorities, who worked closely with Richard Bandler, the founder and developer of NLP. To my surprise, I found that Garner was already doing a lot of work with people who had cancer and so I made an appointment to meet him. Somewhere in my mind I decided that this would be amazing or useless – nothing in between! I was in no state for compromise, I needed help fast. Fortunately for me it did not turn out to be useless – I found 'amazing' instead!

Garner Thomson is a communications specialist and therapist in private practice who, with the support and encouragement of Richard Bandler, has created Medical NLP, the only officially recognized licensed system anywhere in the world that is created specifically for the needs of health professionals and their patients and clients.

The best person to explain how Medical NLP works is Garner Thomson himself, and the following extract is taken from The Middlesex Hospital Chapel Memorial Lecture, which he gave in 1998.

> Medical NLP (as opposed to 'generic' NLP) is specially modelled out of (1) the performance of effective health carers and (2) those clients/patients who heal or recover effectively, sometimes beyond the prognoses given…It is our job as health-care providers (1) to understand the patient/client's map or model of the world, (2) to accept everything that is said as true (rather than impose our own 'meaning' on to his or her experience), then to ask what it could be true of, or how this 'truth' is experienced and is held in place. And, finally (3) to enter that model and help expand or retrieve the possibilities from the inside out … When the doctor or therapist truly recognizes that the map is not the territory (not even when it is our own, passionately defended, medical/therapeutic map), we can congruently and effectively help our patients and clients to create newer, richer and infinitely more useful maps they can use to navigate their way through the challenges and complexities of life.[1]

Based in the UK, Garner Thomson is Training Director for The

Society of Medical NLP, and trains consultants, general practitioners, medical students and ancillary health professionals in the clinical applications of Medical NLP. He is a gentle guy, with a huge love for his work and the people he works with. From the minute we began talking, I felt he was steering a subtle and understanding path. His research at the time stemmed from his realization that patients got better quicker under the care of certain doctors and nurses, and as a consequence of modelling 'the difference that makes a difference', his Medical NLP courses are proving popular in the medical profession. I found it uplifting to know that many doctors are now eager to acknowledge the great value of Medical NLP and want to incorporate it in their practice.

Integration

He then went on to describe how it worked. It seems that those who live a long life tend to take charge of their lives with a good attitude – they 'rise above' things when the going gets tough and are not to be found rigidly doing only the 'right' things. It is now widely acknowledged that the brain affects immunology and vice versa. NLP is the study of how we influence our neurology through language. Garner describes it as the study of subjective experience. It is definitely *not* positive thinking, which always brings guilt and, as he nicely puts it, is therefore 'New Age Fascism'.

The linguistics, that is the data and how we modulate it, is the essence of NLP, and through the linguistics the body sends the message to us to be 'healthy' or 'ill'. This information goes through all five senses, creating a subjective 'map of reality' with which we navigate our way through external 'reality'. The maps we acquire differ from person to person. If they are sufficiently detailed and appropriate, we function efficiently on a day-to-day basis. If they are limited, physical or emotional suffering results. The key is how we use our senses to create our maps, and how willing we are to change and expand them if they prove limiting. With Medical NLP, for example, cancer patients learn that the cancer is not an invader, but something that they are *dealing* with. This helped me enormously because dealing with a problem in music requires a need to understand, integrate and feel, or nothing beautiful will happen. Integration at all levels – physical, mental, psychological and spiritual – is essential to being healthy.

Central to the effective understanding and practice of Medical NLP is the recognition of the toll caused by overloading the system, physically or emotionally – or, more commonly, both. Garner says, 'there is no doubt any more that when our systems are overloaded, we cease to function efficiently, when overload is reduced, we have a much better chance of self-regulating and integrating a more life-directed way of functioning. It's just the way all living things function.'

The big split

One of the greatest difficulties to beset humanity in our modern world is the lack of integration at both the personal and collective levels. As a consequence we have lost our connection with the earth and the cosmos. Moreover, we have become fearful of death. At the collective level, it is not just our relationship with the cosmos that has suffered, but also the relationships between men and women, and between nations, resulting in widespread violence, disruption and destruction. Speaking about the latter to the Study Society in London in January 2004, Ann Baring said that the last 400 years had not recognized the universe as 'conscious'. But this state of affairs in now changing, with scientists gaining a better understanding of consciousness and recognizing that the Universe is indeed conscious. There is also a growing recognition of the relationship between consciousness and energy, confirming what spiritual teachers have been telling us for centuries: we are all connected at a 'quantum' level. In spite of recent advances in our understanding of the 'wholeness' of the universe, however, the influence of scientific materialism still dominates our thinking at both the personal and collective levels in that we tend to split things into ever smaller parts rather then recognizing that they are individual facets of the integrated whole.

NLP master practitioner Nancy Blake wrote about her education, and how she had a problem with what she saw as a 'split' in it.

> ... mathematics and science were opposed to 'soft' topics: literature, languages, and social studies. Psychology was split, with clinical and experimental psychologists in separate warring camps. Freud or Eysenck, psychodynamic theories or behaviourism: there was no common ground; you believed one or the other...In the early 1900s, the idea that mind and body were entirely separate from one another was supported by research which used the inability of large molecules of dye to cross the brain to confirm the 'brain-blood' barrier. In the second half of the last century, however, researchers had demonstrated that certain chemicals, secreted by the glands, interacted not only with other organs, but also with cells in the hypothalamus, the part of the brain associated with the emotions, and with regulation of responses.[2]

She goes on to talk about the great Dr Candace Pert, neuroscientist at the Department of Physiology and Biophysics at Georgetown University Medical Centre, Washington DC, whom Garner Thomson regards as a ground breaker and an inspiration. In her book *Molecules of Emotion*, Dr Pert describes how a similar 'split' affected our understanding of the relationship between mind and body – until more recently, when it became clear that a chemical mechanism existed through which:

> ... the immune system could communicate not only with the endocrine system but with the nervous system and the brain as well. Previous work my colleagues and I had done demonstrated quite convincingly that the brain

communicated with many other bodily systems. But the
immune system had always been considered separate
from the other systems. Now we had definite proof that
this was not the case.[3]

Reintegrating

When Garner speaks of how the immune system misses picking
something up, it is often something personal that is being missed.
The solution is not to go into 'overkill', with drugs and treatments,
but to integrate to regain the balance of immunity. This was to be
confirmed to me later from another direction, during my treatment
with Dr Fryda. I was talking to her about medicine being used
simply to put a part of the body 'right'. She felt that this approach
was wrong and her response was, 'You don't flog a horse when it is
down, do you?' Her approach to physical healing is a subtle one,
and she uses medicine accordingly. In the context of NLP, you don't
bombard the body to 'get the immune system up at all costs' when
it is down, but begin by asking: 'Do you have a sense of connected-
ness in life? Do you want to live? What for?'

It seems that much of the solution is in finding the balance – in
the case of women with breast cancer, a balance between living for
themselves and not overnurturing. As Garner points out, women
are *expected* to play the nurturing role. At an evolutionary level,
men are the ones who go into flight or fight; whereas women go
into fight or appeasement, being better equipped to evolve by
keeping the 'nest' alive.

If we are presented with a situation to which we cannot respond
by fighting or appeasing, we go into lockout or freeze. The trauma
then enters the nervous system and unless it is discharged it causes
dysfunction, usually in the form of depression, or alcohol or drug
abuse. However, evolution has provided us with a safety system
whereby opiates protect the body when it freezes in trauma, as in
the animal kingdom where it protects an animal from a predator by
literally 'freezing' it in its tracks. If the animal escapes the predator,

after a while it will start to shake with relief, then walk away. This is an example of a healthy discharge of trauma, and we cannot hope to balance our body's systems unless we too are able to discharge our traumas.

Nowadays, we are all living with an overload of traumas caused by the speed of living, the environment, toxins and stress, so it is essential to discharge and rebalance ourselves. In the bigger picture, evolutionary advances take place when individual species are faced with a new challenge – for example, the coming of an ice age. Species that do not adapt and rebalance themselves when there is a change in circumstances struggle to survive before becoming extinct. Faced with a new challenge at an individual level, we have a choice of either becoming dysfunctional, or moving up a gear and rebalancing at a higher level.

It is the rebalancing of our physical body (homeostasis) together with the rebalancing of the whole of our being (allostasis) that will, given the right circumstances, allow everyone to correct any previous dysfunction. In order to facilitate this I was given the task of sitting for 15 minutes twice a day, practising a simple mental exercise (not to be confused with a relaxation exercise), as a great way to discharge. It was during one of these 15-minute sessions that I saw the climbing boots, so I asked Garner to explain this to me.

It seems that when an image like this appears, it can be symptomatic of an increase in intuition and a broadening of the sensory range. When we are meditating, the frequency of our brainwaves tends to be between five and nine cycles per second, close to the range of the resonance of the earth, and it is then that the normal blocks of communication drop away. It creates a process that searches out the best for us at certain balance points. Unconscious language doesn't work like our conscious language, often communicating with crazy, irrational images, and, like the incident of my climbing boots, usually indicates something in the future which will only be recognized at the appropriate moment. This 'abstract' part of the brain belongs in the non-dominant hemisphere, whereas 'reality' resides in the dominant hemisphere. It is in the interaction between the two that our health lies.

Many people, ill or healthy, have transformed their lives through using Medical NLP, and if you feel that this is a pathway that could help you, I suggest you try it. You may find that it improves the quality of your life more than you expect.

19 After Surgery – Retail Angels

Every man, woman and child in the world will surely celebrate the day when all the companies who cater for the aftermath of lumpectomies and mastectomies and their retail outlets finally go out of business. This will mean that humanity and science have progressed to the point of abolishing breast surgery as a treatment for disease. Mastectomies and lumpectomies will be a thing of the past. Wishful thinking? It can't come fast enough. Meanwhile…

Lingerie night at Breast Cancer Haven: October 2003

An invitation to a lingerie evening seemed a wonderful diversion as lingerie becomes something of an issue when you have breast cancer, especially if you have not had a reconstruction. This event took place at Breast Cancer Haven in London and the big attraction was to see some of the most beautiful lingerie currently available. To many of us it was a relief that we were going to see real goodies instead of a solemn collection of mastectomy bras which would have been far from 'uplifting' to the spirit.

The show, which was a charity event to raise funds for Breast Cancer Haven, was given by Sheen Uncovered, a lingerie shop in

Sheen High Street, near Richmond-on-Thames, south London. The main reception area of The Haven was turned into a catwalk for the night and the event proved to be a stunning success, not only in raising a considerable sum of money, but by presenting us with glamorous-looking lingerie that 'normal' women would wear. Afterwards, I met the owners of Sheen Uncovered, Anita and Jackie, who said they would be willing to talk to me about their experiences in dealing with women who had breast cancer, and how they can help them.

A visit to Sheen Uncovered

I made an appointment to visit them at their shop, and turned up on a damp, dark November afternoon. In the window I saw lingerie that I had abandoned since surgery, believing that I could only wear normal lingerie after having a reconstruction. I was soon to be proved wrong.

Qualified and experienced in many areas, including maternity and mastectomy, Anita and Jackie keep closely in touch with developments in the lingerie industry. Their warmth was immediate, and over a cup of tea I found out how they deal with women seeking their advice, whether young or old, with or without physical problems. Most important of all, their sensitivity and passion for their work was evident and it became clear that they were much more than mere 'bra-fitters'. Knowing that each person walking into their shop will have a different agenda, they made it clear that breast cancer clients were treated the same as other women.

The treatment of women: surgeons and radiotherapy

Both Anita and Jackie acknowledged that women were in deep trauma when they found they had breast cancer and that several women could go to the same surgeon and yet process the information given to them completely differently depending on the personality of the woman. Jackie had come to the conclusion that surgeons were not the best at putting over the information a woman needed. From her experience, the surgeons were more like mechanics – technical experts – which did not make it any easier for a woman at this very frightening time. They did not claim to pass judgement on the effects of breast cancer treatments on their clients, but when I told them that I had seen some unpleasant results of radiotherapy, they acknowledged that some women appeared to be more severely affected than others.

They talked about the poor quality of breast reconstructions in the past, but noticed that in the previous year or two they had seen some 'very good' and 'incredibly good' ones, largely because one of their local hospitals had a particularly good breast surgeon. The improvement in women receiving nipple replacement was something comparatively new, happening over the previous two to four years.

An emotional issue

Emotionally, breast cancer seemed to be a minefield, and some women were very bitter, often as the result of a particularly bad experience with their treatment. These women were only too eager to seek the experience and understanding of Anita and Jackie, something that neither of them felt was right as it went way beyond their responsibility, as women really required help from the medical establishment. As they pointed out, they are bra-fitters, not doctors, and they feel that their job is to support the women and help them make the best of their appearance. Anita and Jackie saw women trying to deal with their sexuality, body image, post-operation trauma and information overload, all at once. Yet despite the huge ordeal, they found that given time, the tendency is for many women to readjust.

Breast cancer: a grieving process

They observed that through the stages of pre-operation, operation and post-operation, a woman goes through a grieving process. This can cause all kinds of problems, and often a previously friendly woman can become quite difficult and remote. Often she becomes very negative, withdrawn, bitter and aggressive, a state followed by a sudden, almost overnight change when she becomes aware that she is going to survive. Women do this at different times, but it seems to be a process that has to be gone through. Both Anita and Jackie felt that it was at this moment of moving on that the client could be of most help to other women in the same position, but unfortunately by then they no longer required the help of places such as Breast Cancer Haven, which give women such great support, and so generally failed to pass on their own realizations.

The prosthesis

Following a mastectomy, all women are entitled by the NHS to receive a prosthesis which will be supplied by one of a number of selected companies, so the choice is limited. Finding the correct weight of prosthesis is important and here again your choice is limited by the supplier. There are solutions to be had however, just so long as you have an expert who is totally understanding of your needs. As far as Jackie and Anita are concerned, if the client is properly measured and fitted, a prosthesis should be perfectly secure in a normal bra.

Get fitted before the operation

They have offered advice to many breast care nurses who visit them. The nurses can then encourage their patients to visit the shop before they are operated on. This way, Jackie and Anita can follow through the whole process, taking note of the size before the operation, providing suitable soft support immediately after the operation and later dealing with post-operative fitting –

whether it is for a mastectomy, lumpectomy or reconstruction. Although they keep mastectomy bras, they find that very few clients buy these; if the prosthesis is right and you are well fitted, there is no need.

Preferring to be without a prosthesis

I can appreciate women preferring not to wear a prosthesis; some women find that it not only feels uncomfortable but it also feels false and they don't believe they are 'being themselves'. Also, wearing a non-porous, silicone prosthesis next to the skin seems unnatural. Anita and Jackie have fitted women without a prosthesis with a preformed cup, especially for swimming, which many of these women prefer. If you do prefer to be without a prosthesis, finding suitable clothes can be a challenge, but extremely satisfying if you are successful.

Women's vulnerability

It is not difficult to understand the apprehension a woman feels when revealing her scars. Jackie and Anita said that a woman will often turn to them at the crucial moment of baring her body saying, 'Are you ready for this?' Naturally, they are not disturbed at seeing scars or the absence of a breast. Once the client realizes this they quickly settle into the process, although some women just don't like seeing themselves in the mirror and find it difficult. It highlights how incredibly vulnerable we feel having lost a breast.

Whether they are fitting lumpectomy or mastectomy clients, Jackie and Anita find that everybody is different, but they commented that it was easier to fit double mastectomies – whether women have had a reconstruction or not – because they are an even shape. (It is a worrying thought that double mastectomies might be performed for aesthetic reasons). I told them that before meeting them, I would have walked straight past their shop feeling that it was not for me – at least until after a reconstruction. They pointed out that they try to make women feel good about themselves, and that every woman has this right, regardless of circumstances.

Self-image

It is common knowledge in the lingerie business that over 70 per cent of the female population wears the wrong size of bra and that a lot of women believe there is something physically wrong with them when they have difficulty getting a bra to fit. Anita and Jackie say that women simply need expert advice, which is essential when our body image is such a tremendously important matter. Many self-image problems for those with breast cancer have been helped by breast reconstruction work, which in turn has been helped by the ever increasing market for cosmetic surgery and its constantly improving techniques.

But not all those who work in the lingerie business are as sensitive to our needs as Jackie and Anita. My worst experience by far came quite soon after surgery when I was trying to find a bikini in a very smart shop in London's West End. There were two assistants and one or two customers in the shop. The younger assistant came forward and asked if she could help me. Quietly, I told her that I would like a bikini for a mastectomy. Immediately she walked to the long rail of attractive swimwear and ran her hand along the display, looking and saying in a voice loud enough for the whole shop to hear, 'Right, let's see … a *mastectomy* bikini,' with a loud emphasis on the word 'mastectomy'. Horrified, I turned to her and said, 'You don't have to say that so loudly, I don't need the whole shop to know!' Rather than apologize, she then tried to defend herself, but I left the shop during her self-justification, upset at her incredible insensitivity.

We all need to keep a sense of humour – often it is the one thing that really keeps us going. But laughing and trying to brush off other peoples' insensitivity doesn't serve us women. In the long run maybe part of the problem for the appallingly slow progress in breast cancer treatment is the fact that women in general tend to be philosophical and appeasing, often trying to apply a sense of humour when really it would be more appropriate for us to be assertive.

After storming out of the shop, I wrote a letter of complaint to the managing director, to which I got an apology saying that they were looking into the matter. I can only hope that speaking out against poor service will improve things for those who follow. For it is only by speaking out when necessary rather than biting one's tongue, not wanting to rock the boat, or accepting that this is simply 'how things are', that we have the possibility of changing people's attitudes for the better. Putting the incident behind me, I resorted to the mastectomy catalogues, and to my pleasant surprise purchased a very attractive bikini.

Mastectomy wear companies

It appears that very many women find that the prosthesis supplied by their hospital is too heavy and seek a lighter-weight one which is more comfortable. Hospitals tend to point out that the light-weight prostheses are bad for posture, the heavier ones being nearer to the weight of a natural breast. However, I suspect that the effect of an externally applied prosthesis – supposedly the 'correct' weight – is very different from that of a real breast which is supported within our own body structure. Comfort is paramount and each woman is an individual; the idea of there being a standard weight for a breast is just another instance of 'one size fits all'.

There have been great improvements in what the mastectomy companies have to offer to women who've had a mastectomy or lumpectomy (*see* Useful Contacts, pages 253 and 254). The lingerie is vastly improved with a lot of the swimwear just as attractive as normal swimwear, and the styling has advanced enormously. One particular company – Amoena – also issues a quarterly magazine which provides an extraordinary platform for women to write in and share their experiences. The magazine has expanded over recent years with some of the information and research provided by the readers being so important and helpful that the medical establishment would do well to take note. Here you find stories of what really happens when women have had breast surgery, reconstructions and other treatments: those who regard themselves as lucky, those who have had a difficult time and those who find themselves with more cancer. It is not light reading and highlights the deep trauma, bravery and tenacity of all women with breast cancer.

Those working in the mastectomy-wear businesses are well aware of the grim reality. On a daily basis they see women who have undergone some form of breast surgery, usually lumpectomies or mastectomies. Many women frequently describe their horror stories, the self-esteem of a lot of them at zero. Although there are some good reconstructions, it is clear that there are an enormous number of bad ones, some of these so bad that they can make a woman look deformed. It is not uncommon to find a husband who won't look at his wife's scars, and as a consequence many of these women resort to wearing a bra and prosthesis in bed.

For many women, visiting one of these mastectomy-wear outlets may be their first chance to really talk about their feelings. The women who work in these places are remarkable and the service they provide is way beyond their 'job description'. Like Anita and Jackie, they present an opportunity for a woman to begin to regain her self-confidence and her femininity. It says a lot about the way in which women with breast cancer are treated in our health system.

20 The Return – Life After Breast Cancer

Happiness shouldn't be a goal. It isn't something you can achieve, it is the by-product of what you do. What you need to do if you want to be happy is value and accept yourself.

Dr Dorothy Rowe

Like the story told in the first part of this book, my return to wellness and normality has been a continual unfolding of choices. To resume the former life I had before breast cancer was not possible as the world of before seemed different now. So slowly and steadily a new route was created.

Rather like peeling away the layers of an onion, there were small incidents which, rather than alerting me to new moves which I might need to make, were more of a retrospective acknowledgement that I had 'moved on'. During the first three years perhaps the most noticeable of these incidents were those I experienced when returning to Germany for my annual check-ups. On arriving at the airport it was as if a hidden notebook emerged from somewhere in my subconscious, reminding me in a flash of how it had felt to be in the airport the year before. These moments were like putting down markers, signifying weeks or, in this case, months at a time, where some action or thought suddenly jolted me into the realization that things were much better, I was much stronger, and that indeed, I had moved on.

I have often marvelled at the capacity of human beings to deal with the really tough times in life. Over the years I have noticed how friends and colleagues might suddenly run into a crisis, maybe a death in the family, a divorce or separation or other circumstances which caused a major disruption in their lives. Whatever the trauma they had to deal with, when the crisis was over and they finally returned to normal, they seemed stronger in some way. Many years ago, I likewise noticed with fascination how my students – when faced with such circumstances – would eventually return, their voices much more beautiful than before.

Perhaps coming to the end of a tough period with regard to our health is therefore similar, a time to allow the subconscious marker to remind us that things are silently moving forwards and actually, we are all right. It is as if there is a watchful eye monitoring our return to wholeness. The more we can connect with that, the more we acknowledge and reinforce our wholeness.

At another level, the necessary physical caution and self-protection during the early part of my return to health eventually became irksome. To move on, I needed to strengthen my body, but to achieve this wasn't without its problems.

Reclaiming your body

I found that one of the most difficult things to deal with in the aftermath of breast cancer was a strange kind of physical disempowerment. Other women experience a similar feeling. I believe this partly comes about after the operation, when we are told that, from now on, we mustn't lift anything heavy with the arm from which the nodes have been removed. In addition, we are warned that if we get a hangnail – or, heaven forbid, an accidental nick or cut on the hand – we run the risk of setting up an infection and causing lymphodoema (swelling), assuming that it hasn't already arrived in the arm or hand. This was one of the major reasons why I decided not to undergo radiotherapy – along with the fact that I might never again be able to bare my chest to the sun. Of those women who have had radiotherapy, although the risk is greater, not every one will get lymphodoema, whilst others can find it an ongoing problem, some needing to wear an elastic sleeve for much or all of the time. A few women, who have little risk of lympho-doema, wear the sleeve regardless, as insurance. In order to maintain the health of this area of the body, I increased my Tai Chi sessions.

The benefit of exercise

Tai Chi is a good way of gently exercising the body, for it encourages quiet, controlled movement, which is just what you need at this time. A good teacher will be able to set you up with additional exercises to do whilst sitting in bed if you are not able to move very much, gradually progressing further when you are ready. This form of exercise works with the subtle meridians of the body in a similar way to acupuncture, which is also a great healer. Both approaches help balance the system, moving the energy around and often bringing relief from pain.

Tai Chi exercises require a subtle approach, which allows the body to gently start to bloom again. The best way to do this is by regular sessions lasting only a few minutes to begin with, building up to whatever feels comfortable. As it is a moving meditation, you are helping yourself on inner levels whilst at the same time becoming very aware of your body. Take the movements to where you know you are helping the body restore itself, without pushing. Later on, I found Julie Friedeberger's book *A Visible Wound*, very helpful for arm exercises.

Like many women, I suffered numbness behind and under the

upper arm, extending round to the armpit where some of the nodes had been removed. It took almost three years for some feeling to return, which shows how deeply breast surgery affects the body. One doctor suggested that the physical recovery from surgery is quick, and that it is the psychological recovery which can take time. Most women that I have spoken to would disagree with this. Also this suggestion doesn't take into account the additional trauma that the body will endure due to further treatments.

General aches and pains

Every ache and pain is a worry and rings alarm bells in a woman who has had breast cancer. After 14 months I acquired a 'trigger thumb' on the hand of my operation side. This is a painful condition causing a nodule to form and making hand function difficult; as a pianist it worried me that there could be possible consequences from this later on. Just as I was about to put pen to paper and write this book, I found that writing was quite painful and difficult. I sought advice from a hand specialist who recommended cortisone injections, which I refused. A little ultrasound made no difference, and in the end it required time, patience and a supplement of omega 3 to ease the problem. I was relieved to find that having difficulty with joints, particularly the thumb, appears to be a quite common problem in menopausal women, my acupuncturist treating two or three others at that time. Knowing that it was not a problem related to the cancer was good news, but it made me wonder if it was a weakness exacerbated by the removal of the lymph nodes.

Letting go

I found that letting go was a gradual process that couldn't be rushed. After 14 months, I desperately wanted to play tennis again and foolishly indulged in an intensive burst of tennis coaching sessions which left me with tennis elbow, a pianist's nightmare, and something that had never been a problem before. It took a longer time to repair than I had expected. Eventually, after two and a half years, I became very aware that I had done all the sensible things that I had been told to do: Tom had lifted anything that was heavy, whilst I paid great attention to wearing rubber gloves for most household jobs. But things were not feeling right. I felt that I was 'holding on to myself' – the only way I can describe it. I had restricted my movements, had a few aches and pains and realized that I was getting in and out of the car rather too slowly and carefully. Once I became fully aware of this, I knew it was time to do something about it.

With the help of Garner Thomson and his Medical NLP work, I recognized the need to reintegrate a part of myself that had become highly self-protective. I instinctively knew that I had to decrease this intense need for self-protection to a level that was more 'normal'. The transition was quickly and effortlessly achieved and felt like a further homecoming.

The benefits of working out

In her book *Passage to Power*, Leslie Kenton enthuses about the benefits of working out with weights and this appealed to me – after all, I didn't have lymphodoema and could see nothing to stop me. I sought advice from my reflexologist Tony Porter on how to find a good gym and he came up with a suggestion. It was to be the most expensive luxury I gave myself as I planned a routine of working in the gym with a personal trainer twice a week for a year.

A good trainer has probably got a better understanding of the body's motor system than most people and I realized only too well the pitfalls of not using the body well. Two of the younger instructors, Joanna and Daniel, eventually took my sessions, with Daniel ultimately becoming my trainer. On my first visit I was given a thorough check-up, including blood pressure and strength levels, and was quite stunned at my lack of energy which turned into huge fatigue when, far from actually exercising on a machine, I was simply being introduced to it! Rescue came when I remembered that my car was about to run out of time on the meter, which meant that I had to disappear for five minutes to move it, thankful for any opportunity of a break. What a reintroduction to myself. Physically I felt as if I had been on some back burner for years and knew that even with all the self-discipline in the world, I badly needed a helping hand.

Six months later I felt amazingly different. Not only had the aches and pains gone and my energy levels risen, but I was lifting weights which would not have been remotely possible before. I also had the unexpected bonus of my slightly swollen armpit returning to normal. The months of working out achieved all that I had set out to do and more. I no longer got in and out of the car tentatively, I became happy to run without fear, and found no difficulty in picking up a heavy object, Tom having learnt to let me get on with it. Above all, my fitness level rose way above what it had been before the breast cancer, which does wonders for the mind, not only in promoting a healthy outlook, but also in bringing much more confidence. At last, with the help and encouragement of Daniel, I felt that I had totally reclaimed my body.

Strong of body – strong of mind

Somehow, if we feel strong physically, we feel better in our mind. It also works the other way around. I would suggest you do whatever feels comfortable and right for you, and from time to time set out to do something to move yourself on, both physically and mentally. It is part of the holistic process of healing. When we have experienced a trauma such as cancer, we need to listen especially carefully to our needs. If we see problems and we think we know what might help, we should not hesitate to seek out those who will encourage and assist us.

Loyal loved ones

It is not only when we have cancer, but also at other times of crisis that we find out who our true friends and supporters are. Sometimes, when members of the close family and friends cannot cope with the situation, they close themselves off, and this apparently selfish attitude can be devastating. Although particularly hard and hurtful, it's never worth getting into a state about this, because it's simply a decision they take for themselves rather than for you. Don't waste time, the sooner you put it behind you the better. Those who are truly there for you are the ones who, through thick and thin, will be around when you feel up, down, or just plain pissed off. Given time, the result is often a much fuller and richer relationship than ever before, and you gain a greater ability to discriminate in future relationships.

Don't blame yourself

When I was talking about breast cancer to an acquaintance, he shrugged his shoulders and said, 'Well, this breast cancer has been ongoing for years; it's all this cosmetic surgery and implants that cause it.' If only it were so simple. I tried to put him straight, but he seemed indifferent. Those of us who have had breast cancer know only too well that many women with very similar lifestyles to our own will not get breast cancer, and therefore follow this with a bizarre kind of reasoning: if we have breast cancer, it's either because we've omitted to do something to avoid it, or because we've done something 'wrong'. In other words, it's our own fault. This sort of negative reasoning is widespread, and very damaging for women with breast cancer. In this book I have explored some of the many valid reasons why women (and an increasing number of men) get breast cancer, and I hope that the last thing readers who have, or have had breast cancer will be doing is blaming themselves for it. Dr Samuel Epstein (see page 197), has constantly spoken out against the 'blame the victim' syndrome.

Healing

Healing can be extraordinarily beneficial, and Tom (a recognized healer) played a significant part in my journey back to health. But not all encounters are so positive and you need to feel comfortable with the person giving the healing. Unfortunately I met the 'what do you think you have done to bring this on?' syndrome on more than one occasion and wondered if I needed a certificate of proof to say that my cancer was the result of environmental toxins or some such thing. I wonder if this answer would have satisfied those concerned and stopped their 'blame the victim' attitude? The use of amateur psychology can be dangerous and is certainly not appropriate in healing. Good healers have no cause to use it. A healer's job is to heal, not blame. (See Useful Contacts.)

Get in touch with sensation and put your life in order

One of the most useful things we can do after breast cancer is to put the day-to-day running of our life in order. The fragmented state in which so many of us live due to the increased pressure in our lives needs to be addressed, and in many cases brought to a halt. The 2005 BBC2 programmes *Speed Up, Slow Down* highlighted the importance of not running our life on adrenaline and making time and space for ourselves. Once we have achieved this, we can begin to examine the finer details of our lives. I will sometimes teach a student a meditation technique. Contrary to popular belief, meditation doesn't always have to be done with our eyes closed and, with guidance, a similar result can be achieved through vocal exercises. If we practise regularly, we not only become more bodily, but also psychologically aware, and as a consequence can better understand our real needs.

Forward into full health

Now is a perfect time to seek out things that enrich you in ways you would not have otherwise envisaged. Find those things that inspire you and uplift your soul and allow them to become an integral part of your life.

Like countless others, from my earliest childhood I have experienced the sublime joy of listening to fine musicians making music.

Vladimir Horowitz was one of our greatest pianists of the 20th century, and in his eighties was still giving concerts alone onstage to hundreds and thousands of people. Like many of our greatest musicians, he was a particularly sensitive human being. To reach out to an audience and enable them to fly into worlds of sheer, exquisite beauty, elevating us to the opposite end of the spectrum from the mundane, requires huge physical, mental, psychological and spiritual sensitivity. It heals us back into the wholeness from where we can witness the essence of our existence, and when we are privileged to be a part of such an experience, our souls are touched and we are reminded of why we are here.

If, first and foremost, we all choose to become immeasurably loving and generous with ourselves, an enormous potential for healing and growth at every level will open up to us, affecting those around us. Science now recognizes this too. Dr Candace Pert reminds us that 'even when we are "stuck" emotionally, fixated on a version of reality that does not serve us well, there is always a bio-chemical potential for change and growth.'[1] This potential for growth and renourishment can be seen all around us every day, in nature, in the old person who recharges their life with a new diversion and in the baby who joyfully creates its first smile. Sometimes our earliest memories of joy can subtly charge us for the rest of our lives. It all reinforces the fact that we can exercise our ability to find the best for ourselves, to fulfil ourselves at every level and achieve wholeness and abundant health. We help create this by our own choosing – simply by choosing to heal.

Notes

Introduction
1   Smith, Gilly, *Tantra and the Tao*, p 14
2   *Evening Standard*, 7 October 2003

Chapter 2 The Fog Descends
1   www.cloudstrust.org
2   Snow, Sheila & Klein, Mali, *Essiac Essentials*, pp 4, 12

Chapter 3 A Treacherous Path
1   *Institute of Complementary Medicine Journal*, January 2004

Chapter 8 Mammography and Radiation
1   *Breast Cancer Relief News Bytes*, January 2004
2   www.cancerscreening.nhs.uk/breastscreen
3   Department of Health Leaflet 28016/Breast Screening, July 2003
4   Sturgeon, Bill, 'Alternatives to Mammograms,' *Senior News*, Vol. 19, No. 10, 5 October 1998 (Humboldt Senior Resource Centre, Eureka, California)
5   *Daily Telegraph*, 27 September 2000
6   Wright, T; McGechan, A, 'Breast cancer: new technologies for risk assessment and diagnosis,' *Molecular Diagnosis, a journal devoted to the understanding of human disease through the clinical application of molecular biology*, March 2003; 7 (1), pp 49–55
7   *The Times*, 2 June 1991, quoted in Kenton, Leslie, *Passage to Power*, p 99
8   www.health-news.co.uk, 7 November 2002
9   Cox, Dr Roger, 'Screening alert for "at risk" women,' BBC Ceefax 9 November 2002
10 BBC News Health, 9 January 2004
11 Since writing this the NRPB has been renamed and is now the Radiation Protection Division of the Health Protection Agency. Its original name has been retained here because people are still unfamiliar with the NRPB in its new guise. Whatever the reasons may be for the frequent renaming of government bodies and agencies, one thing is clear – it creates unnecessary confusion

among the very people these agencies are supposed to serve. (*See* page 164)

12 BBC Ceefax, 12 January 2004

13 Majid, A S; de Paredes, E S; Doherty, R D; Sharma, N R; Salvador, X, 'Missed breast carcinoma: pitfalls and pearls.' The Radiological Society of North America Inc., *Radiographics 2003*, July–August 23:881–95

14 Berrington de Gonzalez, A & Darby, S, 'Risk of Cancer from diagnostic X-rays: estimates for the UK and 14 other countries,' in *The Lancet*, January 2004, pp 363, 345–51

15 BBC Ceefax, 1 September 2004. Original report: Brenner, D J; Elliston, C D, 'Estimated Radiation Risks Potentially Associated with Full-Body CT Screening,' Radiological Society of North America, *Radiology*, September 2004, 232:735–8

16 Sturgeon, Bill, *Senior News*, Vol. 18, No. 10, 7 October 1999

Chapter 9 Tamoxifen and Similar Drugs

1 'Tamoxifen: Questions and Answers' (NCI Fact Sheet 7.16), available on the website of the National Cancer Institute, www.cancer.gov/cancertopics/factsheet/Therapy/tamoxifen

2 Veronesi, U; Maisonneuve, P; Costa, A; Sacchini, V; Maltoni, C; Robertson, C; Rotmensz, N; Boyle, P, 'Prevention of breast cancer with tamoxifen: preliminary findings from the Italian randomised trial among hysterectomised women,' *The Lancet* Vol. 352, 11 July 1998, pp 93–7. Powles, T; Eeles, R; Ashley, S; Easton, D; Chang, J; Dowsett, M; Tidy, A; Viggers, J; Davey, J, 'Interim analysis of the incidence of breast cancer in the Royal Marsden Hospital tamoxifen randomized chemoprevention trial,' *The Lancet*, Vol. 352, 11 July 1998, pp 98–101

3 Sturgeon, Bill, 'Breast Cancer Awareness Month and Tamoxifen,' *Senior News*, 1 October 2000

4 www.healthsquare.com, 23 January 2005

5 BBC Ceefax 10 June 2006, and www.heratrial.com, 14 June 2006

Chapter 10 Other Women's Stories

1 http:/drhgl.tripod.com/scican.htm

Chapter 11 Politics

1 www.wcrf.uk.org

2 Ibid

3 www.cancerpreventionresearch.org.uk/causes.htm

4 *Ecologist*, Vol. 30., No. 7, October 2000, pp 24–8

5 Last, Walter, 'How Scientific Are Orthodox Cancer Treatments?' *Nexus Magazine*, Vol. 11, No. 4, June/July 2004 www.nexusmagazine.com

6 Ibid

7 Ibid

8 Darbre, P D; Pope, G S; Alijarrah, A; Miller, W R; Coldham, N G; Sauer, M J, 'Reply to Robert Golden and Jay Gandy,' *Journal of Applied Toxicology 24*, (4) 2004, pp 299–301

9 'Scientific Cancer Treatment?', http://drhgl.tripod.com.scican.htm

10 *The Shorter Oxford English Dictionary*

11 *Readers Digest Universal Dictionary*

12 Sturgeon, Bill, 'Breast cancer misunderstanding is perpetuated,' *Senior News*, Vol. 24, No. 28, October 2003

13 Saunders, Thomas, *The Boiled Frog Syndrome*, p 43

14 Skolimowski, Dr Henryk, PhD, from a paper presented to the Fourth Eco-Philosophy Conference on Wholeness and Ways of Being Whole, at Dartington Hall, Devon

Chapter 12 The Golden Key – A Systemic Disease

1 Fryda, Dr Waltraut, *Adrenalinmangel als Ursache der Krebsentstehung* (Kunst & Alltag, 1987), *Diagnose Krebs* (Books on Demand GmbH, 2004), available in English as *Diagnosis: Cancer* (Xlibris Corporation, 2006)

2 Ronzio, Robert A, 'Nutritional Support for Adrenal Function', in *American Journal of Natural Medicine*, 1998

3 www.enlighteningtimes.com/nutrition/walter_last.htm, April 2004

4 *British Journal of Cancer*, August 2003

Chapter 13 Our Environment

1 *Ecologist*, Vol. 30, No. 7, October 2000, p 28

2 Senate Document No. 264, released by the US Government in 1936. Source: www.envirodocs.com

3 *Institute for Complementary Medicine Journal*, April 2004

4 *PEX Newsletter*, No. 11, June 2001

5 *Daily Mail*, 5 September 2003

6 *Evening Standard*, 7 October 2003

7 Watterson, Professor Andrew, 'Working in partnership with

healthcare professionals,' presented at the public meeting 'The Cancer Epidemic: causes and prevention,' in Boston, England, 17 March 2001

8 Wilson, Cynthia, 'Chemical Injury as a Women's Health Issue,' in *Our Toxic Times*, Vol. 8, No. 7, September 1997

9 Sexton, Sarah, 'The Reproductive Hazards of Industrial Chemicals, The Politics of Protection,' *The Ecologist*, Vol. 23, No. 6, November/December 1993

10 Darbre, Dr Philippa, 'Pollutants and Breast Cancer – A Scientific Dilemma,' *PEX Newsletter*, No. 11, June 2001, pp 6–7

11 Saunders, Thomas, op. cit., p 90

12 Ibid, p 73

13 Mc Grath, K G 'Evidence against the use of deodorants and anti-perspirants,' *European Journal of Cancer Prevention* 2003 12(6) pp 479–85

14 *What Doctors Don't Tell You*, Vol. 10, No. 7

15 *Evening Standard*, 30 September 2003, p 26

16 Garland, C F; Garland, F C; Gorham, E D, 'Could Sunscreens Increase Melanoma Risk?', *American Journal of Public Health* 82, 4, 1992, pp 614–5. Quoted in Hobday, Dr Richard, *The Healing Sun*, p 49

17 Hobday, Dr Richard, *The Healing Sun*, pp 149, 150

18 Hobday, Dr Richard, in a talk entitled 'Sunlight Therapy,' presented at The Clouds Trust Cancer Seminar, Elsted, West Sussex, 3 April 2004

Chapter 14 Alternatives to Mammography

1 O'Driscoll, D; Warren, R; MacKay, J; Britton, P; Day, N E, 'Screening with breast ultrasound in a population at moderate risk due to family history,' *Journal of Medical Screening*, 2001; 8 (2):106–9

2 Boisserie-Lacroix, M; Ranchon, N, 'Contribution of high resolution breast ultrasonography in the characterization of ambiguous mammograms,' *Gynécologie, obstétrique et fertilité*, February 2002; 30 (2): 147–53

3 Hou, M F; Ou-Yang, F; Chuang, C H; Wang, J Y; Lee, L W; Huang, Y S; Huang, C J; Hsieh, J S; Lai, C S; Lin, S D; Huang, T J, 'Comparison between sonography and mammography for breast cancer diagnosis in oriental women after augmentation mammaplasty,' *Annals of Plastic Surgery*, August 2002; 49 (2): 120–6

4 Sturgeon, Bill, 'Alternatives to Mammograms,' *Senior News*, Vol. 19, No. 10, 5 October 1998

5 Ibid

6 Waldman, Hilary, 'Electric current shows promise as alternative to mammogram,' *The Hartford Courant*. www.skagitpublishing.com/publications/meddir/news

7 Phillips, M; Cataneo, R N; Ditkoff, B A; Fisher, P; Greenberg, J; Gunawardena, R; Kwon, C S; Rahbari-Oskoui, F; Wong, C, 'Volatile markers of breast cancer in the breath,' *The Breast Journal*, Vol. 9, No. 3, 2003, pp 184–91

8 Wright, T; McGechan, A, 'Breast Cancer: new technologies for risk assessment and diagnosis,' *Molecular Diagnosis, a journal devoted to the understanding of human disease through the clinical application of molecular biology*, March 2003; 7 (1): 49–55

9 *The Times*, 23 April 2004

10 Vachon, C M; Kushi, L H; Cerhan, R J; Kuni, C C; Sellars, T A, 'Association of diet and mammographic breast density in the Minnesota breast cancer family cohort,' *Cancer Epidemiology, Biomarkers and Prevention*, a publication of the American Association for Cancer Research co-sponsored by the American Society of Preventive Oncology, February 2000; 9 (2: 151–60)

11 *Institute of Complementary Medicine Journal*, February 2004

12 Personal interview with Dr Eccles, 1 April 2004

Chapter 15 Menopause – Balancing the System

1 Oriah Mountain Dreamer, *The Invitation*, p 2

2 *Sunday Times Style Magazine*, 1 February 2004

3 For example, Noma Complex Homeopathy (see www.complementary-medicine.com)

Chapter 16 Breast Care, Risks and Prevention

1 *What Doctors Don't Tell You*, Vol. 9, No. 7, October 1998

2 *Sunday Times*, 15 February 2004

3 Wright, Celia, *Higher Nature Health News*, Summer 2003

4 Ibid

5 Ibid

6 For standard melatonin supplements, see www.asphalia.co.uk

7 Saunders, Thomas, op. cit., pp 42–3

8 Health and Safety Commission Newsletter No. 151, October 2003

9   HSE Press Release E132:03, 15 July 2003,
    www.hse.gov.uk/press/2003/e03132.htm

10 Hindle, W H (University of South California School of Medicine,
    Los Angeles), 'Hormone alterations in breast cancer: examining the
    hypotheses,' *Medscape-Women's-Health*, 1999 Jan–Feb; 4 (1): 4

11 Nieman, Lynette K, MD & North, David N, Orth. MD (National
    Institute of Child Health and Human Development, Vanderbilt
    University Medical Centre), 'Treatment of adrenal insufficiency is
    balancing of hormones,' *Medline Journal*

12 *Institute of Complementary Medicine Journal*, April 2004

13 *Prescott Courier Newspaper*, Arizona, and
    www.envirodocs.com/common_cancer_causes.htm

14 Kleijnen, Jos; Knipschild, Paul; ter Riet, Gerben; 'Clinical Trials of
    Homeopathy,' *British Medical Journal*, 9 February 1991

15 *Cancer Prevention and Health News*, Vol. 16, Nos. 4 & 5, 2006

Chapter 17 A Holistic View

1   Edwards, Janet, in a talk entitled 'Taking Charge of Your Own
    Recovery from Breast Cancer,' presented at The Clouds Trust
    Cancer Seminar, Elsted, West Sussex, 3 April 2004

2   Deighton, Hilda; Palermo, Gina; Soresi Winter, Dina, *Singing and
    the Etheric Tone*, pp 13–14

3   Assagioli, R, MD, 'Music: Cause of Disease and Healing Agent,' in
    Campbell, Don (editor) *Music: Physician For Times To Come – An
    Anthology*. See also www.synthesiscenter.org/two.html and
    www.sound-remedies.com.alfredtomatis.html

4   Weeks, B, MD, 'The Physician, The Ear and Sacred Music,' in
    Campbell, Don (editor) *Music: Physician For Times To Come – An
    Anthology*

Chapter 18 Medical Neuro-Linguistic Programming (NLP)

1   Thomson, Garner, extracted from The Middlesex Hospital Chapel
    Memorial Lecture, 1998

2   Blake, Nancy, 'Psychoneuroimmunology and NLP,' *Positive Health*,
    Issue 78, July 2002. www.positivehealth.com

3   Pert, Dr Candace, *Molecules of Emotion*, p 164

Chapter 20 The Return – Life After Breast Cancer

1   Pert, Dr Candace B, *Molecules of Emotion*, p 146

Bibliography and Suggestions for Further Reading

Arnot, Dr Bob, *The Breast Cancer Prevention Diet*, New Leaf Publishing Inc, Houston, Texas, 1999

Bays, Brandon, *The Journey*, Thorsons, London, 1999

Bishop, Beata, *A Time To Heal*, Penguin Arkana, London, 1996

Campbell, Don (editor) *Music: Physician For Times To Come – An Anthology*, Quest, The Theosophical Publishing House, Wheaton, Illinois, 1991

Colthurst, Dr James, *Cancer Positive*, Michael O'Mara Books Ltd, London, 2003

Conteras, Francisco, MD, *The Coming Cancer Cure*, Authentic Lifestyle, Milton Keynes, 2003

Dale, Ralph Alan, *The Tao Te Ching*, Watkins Publishing, London, 2005

Day, Phillip, *Cancer: Why We're Still Dying To Know The Truth*, Credence, Tonbridge, 2003

Daniel, Dr Rosy, *Living With Cancer*, Constable and Robinson, London, 2000

Deighton Hilda; Palermo, Gina; Soresi Winter, Dina, *Singing and the Etheric Tone*, Anthroposophic Press, Hudson, New York, 1991

Epstein, S, Steinman D and LeVert, S, *The Breast Cancer Prevention Program*, Simon and Schuster, Macmillan Company, New York, 1998

Estés, Clarissa Pinkola, *Women Who Run With The Wolves*, Random House, London, 1995

Friedeberger, Julie, *A Visible Wound*, Element Books, Shaftesbury, 1996

Fryda, Dr Waltraut, *Adrenalinmangel als Ursache der Krebsentstehung*, Kunst & Alltag, 1987

Biographie – Grenzerfahrungen, Kunst & Alltag, 1998

Diagnose: Krebs, Books on Demand GmbH, 2004 (German edition)

Diagnosis: Cancer, Xlibris Corporation, 2006 (English edition)

Gearin-Tosh, Michael, *Living Proof*, Scribner, London, 2002

Gerson, Dr Max, *A Cancer Therapy*, Station Hill Press, Barry Town, USA ,1995

Hobday, Richard, *The Healing Sun,* Findhorn Press, Scotland, 1999

Holford, Patrick, *Say No To Cancer*, Piatkus, London, 2000

Hunter, Myra, *Your Menopause*, Pandora, London, 1990

Kenton, Leslie, *Passage to Power*, Vermilion, London, 1996

McTaggart, Lynne, *The Cancer Handbook*, Brian Hubbard, London, 2000

Northrup, Dr Christiane, *The Wisdom of the Menopause*, Piatkus, London, 2002

Pert, Candace B, *Molecules of Emotion: Why You Feel the Way You Feel*, Simon and Schuster, London, 1999

Plant, Professor Jane A, *Your Life In Your Hands*, Virgin, London, 2001

Rowe, Dorothy, *Beyond Fear*, HarperCollins, London, 1994

Rushton, Anna A, and Bond, Dr Shirley A, *Natural Progesterone*, Thorsons, London, 1999

Sampson, Val, and Fenlon, Debbie, *The Breast Cancer Book*, Vermilion, London, 2000

Saunders, Thomas *The Boiled Frog Syndrome: Your Health and the Built Environment*, Wiley-Academy, Chichester, 2002

Sherman, Janette D, MD, *Life's Delicate Balance*, Taylor and Francis, New York, 2000

Smith, Gilly, *Tantra and the Tao*, Robinson Publishing Ltd, London, 1996

Snow, Sheila and Klein, Mali, *Essiac Essentials*, New Leaf, Dublin, 1999

Stewart, Maryon, *Beat The Menopause Without HRT*, Headline, London, 1995

Thomson, Garner, *Magic in Practice – Medical NLP: the Language of Healing and Health*, scheduled for publication in 2007

Tolle, Eckhart, *The Power of Now*, Hodder and Stoughton, London, 2001

Video/DVD/CD

Day, Dr Lorraine, *Cancer Doesn't Scare Me Any More*, www.drday.com

What the Bleep Do We Know?, www.thebleep.com, www.thebleep.co.uk

Inner Talk, www.innertalk.co.uk

Useful Contacts

Organizations and Centres

Breast Cancer Haven
Effie Road
London SW6 1TB
Phone: +44 (0)20 7384 0099
www.breastcancerhaven.org.uk

Breast Cancer Haven
37 St Owen Street
Hereford HR1 2JB
Phone: +44 (0) 1432 361061

Clouds Trust
PO Box 30
Liss
Hampshire GU33 7XF
Helpline: +44 (0) 1730 301 162
    (Monday, Wednesday, Friday:
    9am–12pm)
Fax: +44 (0) 1730 301 162
www.cloudstrust.org

The Integrated Medical Centre
43 New Cavendish Street
London W1G 9TH
Phone: +44 (0) 20 7224 5111
www.integratedmed.co.uk
www.drali.com

**Pesticide Action Network UK
    (PEX)**
Eurolink Centre
49 Effra Road
London SW2 1BZ
Phone: +44 (0)20 7274 8895
+44 (0)20 7274 9084
Email: admin@pan-uk.org
www.pan-uk.org

What Doctors Don't Tell You
4 Wallace Road
London N1 2 PG
www.wddty.com

**Women's Environmental
    Network**
PO Box 30626
London E1 1TZ
Phone: +44 (0)20 7481 9004
www.wen.org.uk

**The Kailash Centre of Oriental
Medicine**
7 Newcourt Street
London NW8 7AA
Phone: +44 (0)20 7722 3939
Email: info@kailash.fsnet.co.uk
Website: www.orientalhealing.co.uk

Australia:
**Cancer Information & Support
Society (CISS) Sydney**
www.ciss.org.au

**Natural Therapy Foundation of
Australia** Melbourne
www.cntf.org.au
Email: cntf@netspace.net.au
Phone: +61 (0)3 9740 3977

The Gawler Foundation
Phone: +61 (0)3 5967 1730

Cansurvive is at the Sunshine Coast (Qld)
Email: csurvive@babe.net.au
Phone/Fax: +61 (0)7 5492 6364

Quest for Life Centre
Phone: +61 (0)2 4883 6599

The Cancer Support Association of Western Australia
www.cancersupportwa.org.au

USA:
The Gerson Institute
1572 Second Avenue
San Diego
CA 92101
Phone: +1 (619) 685 5353
Email: info@gerson.org

Therapies, Individual Medical Practitioners and Therapists

The Chiron Clinic (Breast MITI/Thermography)
104 Harley Street
London W1G 7JD
Phone: +44 (0)20 7224 4622
Fax: +44 (0)20 7935 6652
Email: info@chironclinic.com
www.chironclinic.com

Dr Rosy Daniel BSc MBBCh
Integrated Medical Consultant specializing in helping those with cancer to form effective treatment and self-help plans, including the treatment of cancer with the herbal medicine Carctol, Salvestrol and Iscador.
Apthorp Centre, Weston Road
Bath BA1 2XT
Phone: +44 (0) 845 009 3366

Dr Rosy Daniel (Health Creation Cancer Lifeline Kit)
(address as above)
Health Creation Helpline:
+44 (0) 845 009 3366
www.healthcreation.co.uk

Robert Jacobs (Naturopath)
3 Spanish Place
London W1U 3HX
Phone: +44 (0)20 7487 4334
www.scmhealth.com

Medical NLP
The Society of Medical NLP was established to disseminate the principles of NLP as applied specifically in the field of Positive Health.
www.medicalnlp.com

The National Federation of Spiritual Healers
The Old Manor Farm Studio
Church Street
Sunbury-on-Thames
Middlesex TW16 6RG
Phone: +44 (0)1932 983164
Email: office@nfsh.org
www.nfsh.org.uk

NOMA (Complex Homeopathy) Ltd
www.complementary-medicine.com

Marc Salmon MSc (Oriental Herbal Medicine, Homotoxicology and Electroacupuncture diagnosis)
The Garden Clinic
30A Aldridge Road Villas
London W11 1BW
Phone: +44 (0)20 7221 3899
Email: salmontails@aol.com

Dr F Schellander
(Chelation Therapy)
Liongate Clinic
8 Chilston Road
Tunbridge Wells
Kent TN4 9LT
Phone: +44 (0)1892 543535

Saied Shahsavari
Holistic Health Clinic
64 Chester Road
London N19 5BZ
Phone: +44 (0)20 7263 1414

Dr Mostaraf Ali and Dr Wendy Denning
The Integrated Medical Centre
43 New Cavendish Street
London W1G 9TH
Phone: +44 (0)20 7224 5111
www.integratedmed.co.uk
www.drali.com

Germany:
Dr Kaphahn
Email: wkaphahn@web.de
Phone: +49 (0) 89 645164

Denmark:
Joan Lykke
Vegatest and Vegatest Practitioner Trainer
Danpus ApS
Sofienhøjvej 1
DK-2300 Københaven S
Email: danplus@vegatest.dk
        joan@vegatest.dk
Phone: +45 3252 1420

USA:
Dr Peter Holyk (Thermographic Interpreter) Contemporary Health Innovation, Inc.
600 Shumann Drive
Sebastian
Florida 32958
Phone: +1(722) 388 5554

Dr Nellie Yefet
The Spirit Mountain Healing Arts Center
21400 West Dixie Highway
Aventura, Florida 33180
Phone: +1 (305) 933 2360

Journals and Magazines

Amoena Life (twice-yearly magazine from Amoena; for contact address see under 'Suppliers')
Complementary Therapies in Clinical Practice Journal
PO Box 10
Macclesfield SK10 4HW
Cheshire

Ecologist
Unit 18 Chelsea Wharf
15 Lots Road
London SW10 0QJ
www.theecologist.org

Electromagnetic Hazard and Therapy
Simon Best
9 Nine Acres
Midhurst
West Sussex GU29 9EP
Email: simonbest@em-hazard-therapy.com

Health Essentials (the monthly magazine of Higher Nature; for contact address see under 'Suppliers')

The Institute of Complementary Medicine Journal
PO Box 194
London SE16 7QZ
Email: info@i-c-m.org.uk
www.i-c-m.org.uk

Positive Health
Positive Health Publications Ltd
Queen Square
Bristol BS1 4JQ UK
www.positivehealth.com

What Doctors Don't Tell You
4 Wallace Road
London N1 2 PG
www.wddty.com

Suppliers

Amoena (Mastectomy wear and *Amoena Life*, a twice-yearly magazine)
1 Eagle Close
Chandlers Ford
Eastleigh
Hampshire SO53 4NF
Phone: +44 (0) 23 8027 0345
+44 (0) 800 0728 8866 (for a mail order brochure)
Fax: 023 8026 0877
www.amoena.co.uk

Clouds Trust (René Caisse Herbal Tea, also known as Essiac)
PO Box 30
Liss
Hampshire GU33 7XF
www.cloudstrust.org

Roger Coghill (Melatonin supplement)
Coghill Research Laboratories
Medcross Group Lower Race
Pontypool

Torfaen
South Wales NP4 5UH
www.asphalia.co.uk

Cedric Fisher (Essiac)
74, Highbury Road East
St. Annes-on-Sea
Lancashire FY8 2RW
Phone: +44 (0)1253 727706

Higher Nature (Vitamins and supplements, and *Health Essentials* monthly magazine)
Burwash Common
East Sussex TN19 7LX
Phone: +44 (0)870 0664 478 (Nutrition Department)
0800 458 4747 (Orders)
+44 (0)1435 882 880 (Overseas orders)
Fax: 0870 0664 125
Email: sales@higher-nature.co.uk (Queries only)
www.highernature.co.uk

Nicola Jane Ltd (Mastectomy wear; see below for addresses of Nicola Jane shops)
Southern Gate
Terminus Road
Chichester
West Sussex PO19 8SE
Freephone: 0800 018 2121
Overseas: +44 (0)1243 537 300
Fax: +44 (0) 1243 755922
Email: info@nicolajane.com
www.nicolajane.com

Nicola Jane (Mastectomy wear)
7 City Business Centre
Basin Road
Chichester
West Sussex PO19 2DU
Phone: +44 (0) 1243 533 188

Nicola Jane (Mastectomy wear)
150-164 Goswell Road
London EC1V 7DU
Phone: +44 (0) 207 253 7841

Sheen Uncovered (Lingerie)
287 Upper Richmond Road West
East Sheen
London SW14 7QS
Phone:+44 (0)20 8876 9845
Email: info@sheenuncovered.co.uk
www.sheenuncovered.com

France:
Amoena France S.A.
9, rue du Château d'Eau
FR-69410 Champagne au Mont
d'Or
Contact: Pascale Semiao-Rabilloud
Phone: +33 4 7217 0869
Fax: +33 4 7835 6972
Email: AFPASE@amoena.com
www.amoena.fr

Germany:
Amoena GmbH
Kapellenweg 36
D-83064 Raubling
Contact: Frank Heninger
Phone: +49 8035 87 10
Fax: +49 8035 87 15 60
Email: amoena@amoena.com
www.amoena.de

Spain:
Amoena Espana S.L.
Calle Chile nº4,
Edificio Las Américas I, oficina 7
ES – 28290 Las Matas-Madrid
Contact: Paz Martinez
Phone: +34 91 630 84 71
Fax: +34 91 630 01 42
Email: ESPMV@coloplast.com
www.es.amoena.com

Sweden:
Amoena Sweden AB
Sveavägen 52
SE – 11134 Stockholm
Contact: Ingrid Warnelid
Phone: +46 854 525 770
Fax: +46 8 791 88 37
Email: asinfo@amoena.com
www.amoena.se

Canada:
Coloplast Canada Corporation
3300 Ridgeway Drive, Unit 12
CA – Mississauga, Ontario L5L 5Z9
Contact: Voula Pantelis
Phone: +1 905 820 7588
Fax: +1 905 820 0522
Email: cavp@coloplast.com

USA:
Coloplast Corporation – Amoena
US
1701 Barrett Lakes Blvd.
Suite 410
Kennesaw, GA 30144
Contact: Lori Austin-Bunton
Phone: +1 770 281 8300
Fax: +1 800 723 3464
Email: info@amoena.com
www.us.amoena.com or
www.thebreastcaresite.com

Index